Ophthalmic DOPS and OSATS

The handbook for work-based assessments

SAM EVANS

BSc BMBS FRCOphth
ST6 Ophthalmology Registrar
University Hospital of Wales, Cardiff

Foreword by

PATRICK WATTS

MBBS MS FRCS FRCOphth
Consultant Paediatric Ophthalmologist
College Tutor
University Hospital of Wales, Cardiff

D1344450

Radcliffe Publishing
London • New York

Radcliffe Publishing Ltd
St Mark's House
Shepherdess Walk
London N1 7BQ
United Kingdom

www.radcliffehealth.com

British Library Cataloguing in Publication Data
A catalogue record for this book is available from the British Library.

ISBN-13: 978 184619 549 5

The paper used for the text pages of this book is FSC® certified. FSC (The Forest Stewardship Council®) is an international network to promote responsible management of the world's forests.

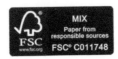

Typeset by Beautiful Words, Auckland, New Zealand
Manufacturing managed by 21six

Contents

Surgical skills   91

Appendix: key studies and guidelines   113

Foreword

The introduction of the European Union Working Time Directive increased public expectations, and the technological advances in medicine called for a change in the way doctors are educated in the workplace. A reduction in the junior doctor's hours, which compromised the time and opportunities for clinical exposure, triggered a change in the model of medical education towards one that is outcome and competency based. Therefore, it is imperative that the opportunities for learning are maximised in a doctor's learning environment. There are 179 competency requirements of the Ophthalmology trainee embedded in The Royal College of Ophthalmologists' training curriculum. This may seem daunting to the trainee with little experience in Ophthalmology in a learning environment that has hitherto been reliant on an apprenticeship model of experiential learning. This book provides the trainee and trainer with lucid explanations of workplace competency requirements. It includes instructions on the techniques of clinical examinations, investigations and methods of undertaking practical procedures, which maps well against the curriculum.

This book is a welcome addition to support the trainee's learning and serves as a useful reference when undertaking assessment either in the workplace or summative evaluations in examinations.

Patrick Watts MBBS MS FRCS FRCOphth
Consultant Paediatric Ophthalmologist
College Tutor
University Hospital of Wales, Cardiff
September 2014

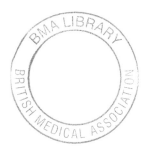

Acknowledgements

I have received endless patient support from many colleagues throughout the writing of this book, whose proof reading and editing has resulted in what I hope is a useful resource for trainees of the future.

In particular I am grateful to Vinod Kumar for his encouragement and enthusiasm in the early stages of writing, and to Patrick Watts for his towards the end.

Patience and wisdom have always been hallmarks of my father's advice to me – this was particularly the case during the writing of this book. For this, and the inspiration to follow him into a career in Ophthalmology, I am indebted to him.

Finally, many thanks to the nursing and orthoptic staff who bravely 'volunteered' themselves as models for the illustrations where patients were not available.

Preface

Ophthalmology is a challenging and rewarding specialty that is underrepresented in undergraduate education. The introduction of The Foundation Programme for early postgraduate training has encouraged the development of generic skills, few of which are applicable to Ophthalmology. Therefore, trainee Ophthalmologists frequently start their training with little or no experience of the practical skills specific to the specialty. Further, Ophthalmology departments are among the busiest in any hospital, meaning that opportunities for direct teaching are limited, and the demand for juniors to undertake procedures is significant. This represents a challenge, to both the trainee and the trainer, to provide an environment in which skills are acquired and honed while patient safety and consistency of technique are maintained.

This book aims to provide the trainee Ophthalmologist with a guide to many of the practical skills which appear on The Royal College of Ophthalmologists' (RCOphth) syllabus. While it is rare nowadays for the trainee to be expected to 'just get on with it' and make their mistakes on the job, the merit of such a guide is as a reference as skills are learned and refined.

A generally consistent format is used throughout the book, with reference to the College syllabus through the use of their codes and target years of achievement. Each skill or technique has an aim, and a list of equipment required when this is appropriate. A bullet-pointed, step-by-step walk-through of the key steps for the skill follow, with specific tips, or 'pearls', when these are important. Line drawings further illustrate techniques. In some cases discussion of the basic principles underlying an investigative technique, or the physiology of a particular sign, is included.

It is important to acknowledge that the specific details herein represent only one way to attain these skills – the trainee should always refer to local practice and take advice from their senior colleagues until they are comfortable undertaking a procedure unaided. While the College curriculum is generally used as a structure for the skills discussed, the contents of this book are not a complete list of the College curriculum – and their inclusion does not imply the approval of The RCOphth.

The Appendix contains a concise summary of 50 major ophthalmic studies and papers, together with a summary of RCOphth and National Institute for Health and Care Excellence and DVLA guidance pertinent to Ophthalmology. Trainees studying for Fellowship of the Royal College of Ophthalmologists (FRCOphth) will find these summaries useful as part of their revision.

I am grateful to those forgiving colleagues who have taught me in the past, those who continue to do so, and those who will do so in the future. Any virtue as may be found in these pages is thanks to their patient tuition. Those errors and omissions that exist are mine.

Sam Evans BSc BMBS FRCOphth
Cardiff
September 2014

About the author

Sam Evans is an Ophthalmology registrar based in South Wales. He trained initially in ecology, before going to medical school in Exeter.

Outside work, he enjoys camping with his children, fly fishing, kitesurfing and paddle boarding.

He has an interest in medical device development and design. In particular, improving the links between clinicians and designers to produce new and effective devices.

He hopes one day to become a lobster fisherman.

List of abbreviations

AHP	abnormal head posture
AL	axial length
ALT	argon-laser trabeculoplasty
AMD	age-related macular degeneration
AP	anteroposterior
BCVA	best-corrected visual acuity
BDR	background diabetic retinopathy
BP	blood pressure
BRVO	branch retinal vein occlusion
BSV	binocular single vision
CCT	central corneal thickness
CJD	Creutzfeldt–Jakob disease
CN	cranial nerve
CNV	choroidal neovascularisation
COAG	chronic open-angle glaucoma
CRAO	central retinal artery occlusion
CRT	central retinal thickness
CRVO	central retinal vein occlusion
CSM	central, steady and maintained
CSMO	clinically significant macular oedema
D	dioptre
DD	disc diameter
EDTs	electrodiagnostic tests
EDW	Edinger–Westphal
EOG	electrooculography
ERG	electroretinography
ETDRS	Early Treatment Diabetic Retinopathy Study
FAZ	foveal avascular zone
FDDT	fluorescein dye disappearance test
FFA	fundus fluorescein angiography
FMT	fluorescein meniscus time
FRCOphth	Fellowship of the Royal College of Ophthalmologists
GC	ganglion cell
GDD	glaucoma drainage device
HRR	Hardy–Rand–Rittler
I-CRVO	ischaemic central retinal vein occlusion
IO	inferior oblique
IOL	intraocular lens
IOP	intraocular pressure
IR	inferior rectus
IV	intravenous
IVTA	intravitreal triamcinolone
KTP	potassium titanyl phosphate
LR	lateral rectus
MGD	meibomian gland dysfunction
MR	medial rectus
MRI	magnetic resonance imaging
MS	multiple sclerosis

nAMD	neovascular age-related macular degeneration
NICE	National Institute for Health and Care Excellence
NI-CRVO	non-ischaemic central retinal vein occlusion
NV	new vessels at the disc
NVA	new vessels at the angle
NVI	new vessels at the iris
OCT	optical coherence tomography
OHT	ocular hypertension
p.o.	*per os*
PDR	proliferative diabetic retinopathy
PDT	photodynamic therapy
POAG	primary open-angle glaucoma
PPDR	pre-proliferative diabetic retinopathy
PRN	*pro re nata*
PRP	pan-retinal photocoagulation
PTN	pre-tectal nuclei
RAPD	relative afferent pupillary defect
RCOphth	The Royal College of Ophthalmologists
RD	retinal detachment
ROP	retinopathy of prematurity
RPE	retinal pigment epithelium
Rx	prescription
SEM	slow eye movement
SITA	Swedish interactive threshold algorithm
SLO	scanning-laser ophthalmoscopy
SLT	selective laser trabeculoplasty
SNR	signal-to-noise ratio
SO	superior oblique
SR	superior rectus
TBUT	tear-film break-up time
UBM	ultrasound biomicroscopy
VA	visual acuity
VAVFC	vigabatrin-attributed visual-field constriction
VEGF	vascular endothelial growth factor
VEP	visual evoked potential
VF	visual field
VMT	vitreo-macular traction
WTW	white-to-white
YAG	yttrium aluminium garnet

Clinical assessment

CODE: CA2
TARGET YEAR: 1

CLINICAL CONTEXT

The assessment of visual acuity (VA) provides the Ophthalmologist with an objective measure of visual function. It is simple to measure and provides a repeatable and consistent indication of central acuity.

BASIC PRINCIPLES

'Acuity measurements' determine the ability of a visual system to differentiate two targets separated by space. Central acuity is generally measured by recognition of optotype charts, although non-literate targets may be used. It is important to recognise that central acuity is only one aspect of visual function.

Acuity measurements are based on the assumption that the foveal cone photoreceptors are able to resolve (differentiate) light subtending an angle of 10 arc minutes (spatial resolution). In fact, significantly higher orders of resolution (greater than 0.5 arc minutes) can be made by the human eye (vernier acuity). This is a product both of intraretinal processing of relative stimulation of neighbouring cones and, to a greater extent, of higher (post-retinal) centres. Vernier acuity is measured using offset gratings, whereas gross acuity is measured by optotype charts.

The ability to resolve a target is affected by its contrast when compared with its background and by the angle subtended at the retina (size of target). Therefore, two acuity-measurement systems may be used:

1 high-contrast – typically black on white – targets of varying size (Snellen, LogMAR and Early Treatment Diabetic Retinopathy Study [ETDRS] charts)
2 varying-contrast targets of uniform size (Pelli–Robson Contrast Sensitivity charts).

Measurements of contrast sensitivity can give an excellent indication of cone function, but consistent inter-test reliability is difficult to achieve.

EQUIPMENT LIST

- Vision chart (Snellen or LogMAR)
- Occluder

PROCEDURE

1 Ensure the patient is at the distance from the chart specified by the chart type:
   ➤ Snellen acuities should be measured from 6 m (with a mirror at 3 m if required)
   ➤ LogMAR acuities are measured from 4 m.
2 Occlude one eye at a time, asking the patient to read down the chart to the smallest line that is clearly visible, encouraging them to continue until they begin to get letters wrong.

The pinhole provides as close as is practical to a single, axial (and, therefore, unrefracted) beam of light. This overcomes ametropic error and should be used when uncorrected acuity is unexpectedly poor.

NOTATION

- By convention, information regarding the right eye is recorded on the left-hand side of the page, and that regarding the left eye on the right, as the examiner sees the patient.
- Uncorrected acuity should be recorded, followed by the best-corrected visual acuity (BCVA) whether by pinhole or formal refractive correction.

Pearls

▸ Snellen acuity is recorded as a fraction, with the numerator recording the distance in metres from the chart and the denominator the distance at which the smallest target (optotype) subtends 5 minutes of arc.

▸ Snellen fractions compare the subject's acuity with that which would be expected at a given distance from the target.

  – Thus, an acuity of 6/60 implies that the eye can only resolve a target from 6 m, whereas a normal eye would see the target at 60 m.

▸ LogMAR acuity is recorded as a decimal on a scale from 0.000 to 1.000, on which 0.000 is equivalent to 6/6 and 1.000 is equivalent to 6/60. Negative LogMAR acuities demonstrate vision better than 6/6.

  – On a LogMAR chart, each letter represents 0.02 LogMAR.

  – LogMAR charts reduce the error caused by the crowding phenomenon and use a logarithmic scale, overcoming the significant jumps in acuity between various points on a Snellen chart.

▸ Ametropic eyes with no other pathology should achieve higher acuities with the use of a pinhole – however, when cataract or other media opacities are present, the pinhole will seldom improve an eye with poor acuity to one with 6/6 vision; nevertheless, an improvement with pinhole should give the surgeon some reassurance that removing the cataract and providing adequate post-operative refraction should result in improved VA.

Assess vision: acuity in children or illiterate adults

> **CODE:** CA2
> **TARGET YEAR:** 1
> **AIM:** to measure the level of resolution of a child's visual system in a reproducible manner.

BACKGROUND

Illiterate adults and children require special acuity-measurement strategies, which must be tailored to the subject's age and literacy.

The eye not being tested should be occluded. This can be done with an amblyopia occlusion patch. However, very young children may object to either eye being covered. In these cases, binocular acuity should then be measured.

INFANTS (PRE-VERBAL; 0–6 MONTHS OLD)

Vision assessment in pre-verbal children is challenging but important. The early detection of reduced vision is important so treatment to prevent the development of amblyopia can be started. The vision of very small infants is initially assessed by observation. The ability of a child to maintain central, steady and maintained (CSM) fixation is an indication of visual function, as is the ability to fix on and follow a target. The target should be bright and the room free of distractions. A child who objects particularly to the occlusion of one eye may have reduced vision in the fellow eye. Forced-choice preferential-looking tests may be used from birth, although their reliability increases as the infant gains head-position control. In young infants, these tests require considerable interpretive skill on the part of the examiner and should be used in conjunction with CSM and clinical observation to build an idea of the probable visual capacity of the child.

Infants older than 18 months may be cooperative with more objective testing.

Equipment list
- Teller Acuity Cards™
- Cardiff Acuity Test™ cards (aged 6 months–3 years old)

Background

VA testing in this group is based on preferential-looking tests. The subject is presented with a board with a single target and a blank area, and the tester observes which area of the card is of interest to the subject. Typically, these tests consist of gratings (Teller) or simple shapes (Cardiff cards) of varying contrast when compared with their background. The tests may be used at varying distances from the subject, with a guide to the likely acuity being provided for each given distance.

Preferential-looking tests are, by nature of the test and the subjects, a coarse measurement of VA.

Procedure

Testing should be carried out in a well-lit room, free from distractions.
1 Sit directly in front of the subject, at the appropriate distance, as indicated on the card.
2 Hold the testing cards face down on your knee.
3 Quickly bring up one card at a time to the subject's eye level, and observe their response through the observation hole in the middle of the card.
4 Recheck an equivocal response by reorientating the card.

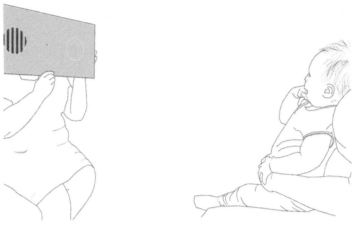

FIGURE CA2.1 Use of Teller Acuity Cards™

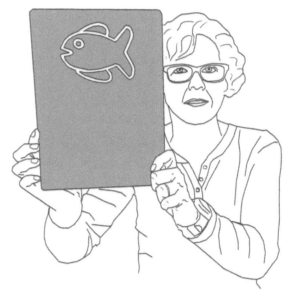

FIGURE CA2.2 Use of Cardiff Acuity Test™ cards

VERBAL CHILDREN (3–4 YEARS OLD) AND ILLITERATE ADULTS
Equipment list
- Kay Picture Test Cards
- Tumbling E chart
- Matching Board

Background
Testing the VA of individuals who are able to recognise and match shapes provides a better indication of acuity resolution than preferential-looking tests. A variety of techniques exist for this group, although each is based on the presentation of targets (shapes or optotypes) of varying contrast or size.

The most commonly used test in this group is the crowded Kay Picture Test. This overcomes some of the overestimation of acuity inherent in single optotype targets by crowding the targets.

Procedure
Testing should be carried out in a well-lit room, free from distractions.
1 Sit directly in front of the subject, at the appropriate distance.
2 Provide the subject with a matching board, with high-resolution examples of each of the targets they will be presented with on a single sheet.
3 Hold the testing cards face down on your knee then present them one at a time to the subject.
4 Ask the subject to indicate on their matching board which shape or letter they can see.

LITERATE CHILDREN (>4 YEARS OLD)
Equipment list
- Snellen chart
- LogMAR chart
- ETDRS chart
- Occluding glasses
- Matching board

Procedure
Test literate children using a standard literate optotype chart. This may be used with a matching card if the child is unsure of letter names.

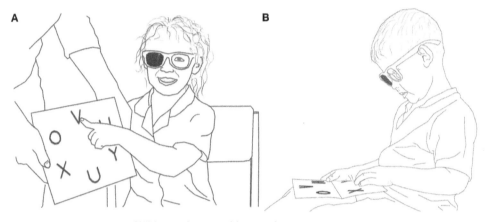

FIGURE CA2.3A AND B Children using matching cards

Pearls
▶ Preferential-looking tests tend to overestimate VA – this is particularly true of amblyopic eyes.
▶ It is of the utmost importance that the testing environment be quiet and free from distraction.
▶ Young children tire quickly and lose motivation. If you are getting nowhere, it may be wise to move on to another part of your assessment, before returning to acuity testing.
▶ A lot of information about a child's acuity can be gathered by simply observing them interacting with their environment.

CODE: CA2
TARGET YEAR: 1

CLINICAL CONTEXT

The perception of colour is a cortical construct built on the stimulation of cone photoreceptors sensitive to specific wavelengths. Considerable intraretinal and cortical processing occurs to construct the colour percept, based on three basic cone photoreceptor types, L, M and S (representing long, medium and short wavelengths, respectively, within the visible spectrum). The differential stimulation of neighbouring photoreceptor populations of different sensitivities gives rise to the perception of hue. Disruption of conduction along the optic nerve will result in disturbances in colour vision, in particular, the saturation of reds. Colour-vision testing is therefore one of the five assessments of optic-nerve health – the remainder being relative afferent pupillary defect (RAPD), visual fields, VA and direct observation of the disc.

EQUIPMENT LIST

- A colour perception chart:
  - ➤ Ishihara pseudo-isochromatic plates for red and green deficiency
  - ➤ Hardy–Rand–Rittler (HRR) test plates for red, green and blue deficiency
  - ➤ The City University Colour Vision Test cards for red, green and blue deficiency
  - ➤ Farnsworth–Munsell 100 Hue Color Vision Test
  - ➤ Farnsworth–Munsell D15 Color Vision Test
- Occluder

PROCEDURE

Ensure test charts are well illuminated, preferably with natural light, and that near refractive correction is worn if appropriate.

Plate tests (Ishihara and HRR)

1 Provide adequate refractive correction.
2 Isolate each eye with an occluder.
3 Ask the patient to read each plate in turn.
  - ➤ If the patient is illiterate, use the patterned plates and ask them to trace along the edge of the swirling pattern.

The City University Colour Vision Test

1 Provide adequate refractive correction.
2 Isolate each eye with an occluder.
3 Show each plate in turn.
4 Ask the subject to choose which dot most closely matches the hue of the central target.

Farnsworth–Munsell 100 Hue Color Vision Test

The test consists of four trays with a total of 85 hues. This is a very long test, which is usually undertaken by the orthoptic team. A shorter screening test (the Farnsworth–Munsell D15 Color Vision Test) is also available.
1 Ask the patient to arrange the hues in order.
2 Compare their results with the correct order to determine their colour perception and aptitude.

Use of the Amsler grid

CODE: CA4
TARGET YEAR: 1

BASIC PRINCIPLES

The spatial relationships of ganglion cells (GCs) within the retina extend first to the lateral geniculate nucleus and then to V1 in the visual cortex. This retinotopic mapping is maintained, even if the position of the GCs is altered. Thus, disturbance in the GC position results in distortion of the perceived image – when GCs are disproportionately separated when compared with their V1 position (i.e. in retinal oedema), the image will appear pinched. Similarly, contraction of the spaces between them (i.e. in retinal fibrosis) causes straight lines to appear bent or curved. This phenomenon of metamorphopsia is assessed using the Amsler grids. These are a family of seven charts based on regular perpendicular gridlines with a central fixation target. Alignment aids are provided on some of the charts for patients with significant central scotomas, and both monochrome and coloured charts are available. It is a screening test, and, in most cases, the chart used is a box grid of black lines on a white background with a black central target.

EQUIPMENT LIST

- Amsler grid

PROCEDURE

This is a uniocular test.

1 Ask the patient to wear their normal refractive correction for near, and cover the fellow eye.
2 Ask them to hold the grid at arm's length and observe the fixation target. Encourage the patient to report any distortion in the grid adjacent to the target. A patient with distortion of the macula will report corresponding distortion of the grid.
3 Ask them to then trace the distorted lines on to the grid.
4 Repeat the test for the fellow eye.

> **Pearl**
>
> ▶ The Amsler grid is most commonly used in the age-related macular degeneration (AMD) clinic where patients may be encouraged to pin a grid up in their house to allow for frequent testing. It is also a useful screening test for many other macular pathologies including epiretinal membrane formation, macular holes and diabetic maculopathy.

BASIC PRINCIPLES
Pupil size is controlled by the muscles of the iris: the sphincter pupillae (circumferential fibres) and the dilator pupillae (radial fibres). Innervation of the sphincter is via parasympathetic fibres from the third-nerve nucleus via the ciliary ganglion and short ciliary nerves. The dilator is innervated by sympathetic fibres from the superior cervical ganglion. The stimulus to contract or dilate the pupil is derived from retinal information regarding incident light and is controlled by an afferent–efferent loop involving receptors (retina), processors (pre-tectal nuclei [PTN] and Edinger–Westphal [EDW] nuclei) and effectors (sphincter pupillae).

The afferent limb decussates at the chiasm, travelling with the optic tract, but bypassing the lateral geniculate body, and entering the PTN and EDW nuclei. As the fibres have decussated, a uniocular stimulus will evoke a bilateral innervation at the level of the PTN and EDW. The efferent limb travels to the sphincter pupillae via the parasympathetic fibres of the third nerve, synapsing in the ciliary ganglion.

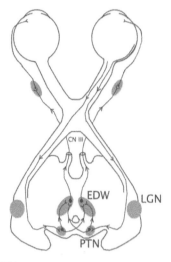

FIGURE CA6.1 Pupillary pathway
Abbreviations: CN, cranial nerve; LGN, lateral geniculate nucleus

CLINICAL APPLICATION
In practical and clinical terms, there are two types of pupillary reflex that are of interest: (1) the light reflex and (2) the near reflex. Accurate examination of these simple signs will garner a depth of information about the neuronal capacity of the anterior visual pathway and inform the direction of subsequent history taking and examination.

LIGHT REFLEX
There are three pupillary light reflexes of interest:
1 the direct response
2 the consensual (afferent) response
3 the relative afferent response.

The direct response is observed on bright illumination of the pupil of the illuminated eye. A reflex constriction demonstrates intact ipsilateral afferent and efferent pathways as well as a functioning retina and sphincter pupillae.

The consensual response is observed as a simultaneous pupillary constriction of the contralateral pupil. This demonstrates an intact afferent pathway on the illuminated side and efferent pathway on the contralateral side, as well as a functioning EDW nucleus.

Impaired afferent function of the optic nerve may be found in inflammatory, infiltrative or compressive lesions of the nerve and is demonstrated by comparing its response with that of its fellow. This is termed a 'relative afferent pupillary defect' (RAPD) and is an important test of optic-nerve function. A difference in direct and consensual constriction suggests impaired afferent function of the affected optic nerve.

EQUIPMENT LIST
- Bright spot illumination (an indirect ophthalmoscope is ideal)
- Near target

NEAR REFLEX
The near reflex forms one-third of the 'near triad' (the other two parts of the triad being lenticular accommodation and convergence) and is a simultaneous symmetrical miosis when the patient is presented with a near target. Failure of the light reflex with an intact near reflex is known as light–near dissociation and is seen in the dorsal midbrain syndrome, neurosyphilis (Argyll Robertson pupil) and degenerative neuropathies.

PROCEDURE
Ensure that the patient has not had mydriatic or miotic agents instilled prior to examination and that they are sitting in a dimly lit room.
1   Ask the patient to fixate on a distance target in order to overcome the miosis associated with the near triad; it is not necessary for the patient to wear refractive correction.
2   Take care to stand away from the visual axis and not to obstruct it with either your hand or a torch.
3   Illuminate one eye with a bright white spot light, noting the immediate response of the pupil (**direct response**).
4   Swing the illumination to the fellow eye, again observing the direct response.
5   Repeat the process, this time observing the un-illuminated eye (**consensual response**).
6   Finally, as you swing the light between each eye again, observe the response of the illuminated eye (**relative afferent response**).
7   To test the **near reflex**, present the patient with a near target (within 33 cm, or an arm's length) while asking them to fixate on a distance target, then ask them to fixate on the near target and observe both pupils.

Pearls
▶ The RAPD is not an 'all-or-nothing' sign; there are varying degrees of penetration, which can be measured using neutral density filters. The density of the defect is usually a fair reflection of the interruption to optic-nerve conduction.
▶ The RAPD is seen in disorders of optic-nerve conduction; therefore, it may be seen in large retinal detachments, central retinal artery occlusion (CRAO), anterior ischaemic optic neuropathy, optic neuritis, end-stage glaucoma, neoplastic infiltration of the optic nerve and compressive lesions affecting the nerve. It is not seen in cataract, primary corneal disease, or early or moderate glaucoma.

CODE: CA7
TARGET YEAR: 2

BASIC PRINCIPLES

Ocular movements consist of:
- versions: bilateral movements in the same direction (conjugate movements)
- vergences: bilateral movements in opposite directions (disconjugate movements)
- ductions: uniocular movement in the horizontal, vertical or torsional plane.

'Versions' are conjugate deviations of gaze (both eyes move in the same direction). They are either fast refixations (saccades) or slow, following movements (smooth pursuit), and are essential for binocular vision. Control of the relative position of each eye during a version is important to avoid diplopia. This is coordinated by the horizontal gaze centre of the paramedian pontine reticular formation, the effect being propagated bilaterally via the medial longitudinal fasciculus, ensuring bilateral stimulation of the yoked horizontal recti. Vertical versions are mediated via the rostral interstitial nucleus of the medial longitudinal fasciculus.

Versions, which are required to follow a target that is moving relative to the eye, may be of two types: (1) slow eye movements (SEMs), required for smooth pursuit of a slowly moving target, and (2) refixation movements (saccades), used for refixation of a rapidly moving target.

SEMs provide uninterrupted pursuit of a target that is moving relative to the eye. Unlike saccadic movements, they require constant adjustment, informed by visual cues, as to the target's velocity and direction or, when the head is moving, proprioceptive feedback. SEMs tend to be more accurate in the horizontal meridian and are almost impossible to undertake without a visual cue. As a result of the complex inter-nuclear communication required for these movements, SEM is impaired in many neurodegenerative conditions.

'Saccadic movements' are refixation movements whose velocity and duration are preset at the time of initiation (ballistic). Their stimuli are visual (from the frontal eye fields), auditory, positional or to command. The speed of refixation is around 900 degrees per second. During this time, the cortex suppresses visual perception to avoid a disorientating smearing of the percept. After the eyes have arrived at the predetermined new position, compensatory microsaccades fine-tune position.

Nystagmus is a combination of both SEM and saccades, and is a useful demonstration of the difference between the two types of movement. The 'drift phase' is a typical SEM that either slips behind or overshoots the target followed by a rapid refixating saccade. The direction of the nystagmus is named after the direction of the fast 'beat' of the saccade, although, in general terms, it is the slow phase that is the pathological component, while the saccade is an attempt to recapture the lost target.

'Vergence' eye movements are bilateral movements in opposite directions. They may be towards the midline (*convergence*) or away from it (*divergence*). They are required to maintain focus on a target moving towards or away from the viewer.

'Ductions' are uniocular movements and are described with respect to the direction of movement in relation to the original position. They may be *ab*duction (away from midline), *ad*duction (towards midline), *infra*duction (downward movement) or *supra*duction (upward).

'Torsional' movements are those which occur along the Z-axis of the eye and can be considered rotatory movements. They may be *incyclotorsion* (rotation towards the midline) or *excyclotorsion* (away from midline). They are chiefly related to the oculocervical reflex and the maintenance of stable vision with head rolling. Their chief effectors are the oblique muscles, although the vertical recti also provide some torsional movement in eccentric positions of gaze.

The effectors of horizontal movements are the medial and lateral recti. The effect of the obliques is predominantly vertical when the eyes are in adduction and torsional when the eyes are in abduction. The vertical recti are responsible for vertical movements when the eyes are in abduction.

Movements should be examined in a position that, as closely as possible, isolates the function of each muscle and, further, where this function is clearly identifiable and specific to the muscle being tested.

It is particularly important to be aware of the torting action of the vertical muscles and avoid testing the muscle in a position where it may exert a torsional effect. For this reason, the superior rectus (SR) should be tested in abduction, when its intorting effect is minimised and inferior rectus in abduction in order to minimise its excyclotorsion in adduction. The superior oblique (SO) has a mixed intorsional and depressor action in the primary position. When tested in adduction, the intorsion is much reduced, and this is the position in which its function is best observed. The inferior oblique should be also be tested in adduction in order to reduce its excyclotorsion effect in the primary position. The failure of the SO to intort in cranial nerve (CN) IV palsy is the basis of Bielschowsky's head-tilt test, as discussed on p. 17.

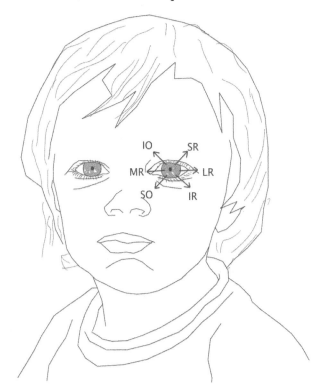

FIGURE CA7.1 Extraocular muscle actions

LAWS OF OCULAR MOVEMENTS

There are two physiological laws that govern the movement of the two eyes:

1 Sherrington's law of reciprocal innervation: the antagonist pair for each eye is reciprocally innervated. Consequently, a stimulus to one of the pair is accompanied by inhibition of the antagonist; this ensures unrestricted action in the intended direction

2 Hering's law of binocular innervation: the stimulus to the yoked muscle of the fellow eye is equal; this ensures stable, comitant movement (this does not apply in vergence movements).

EQUIPMENT LIST
- Target
- Occluder
- Prism bar
- Optokinetic nystagmus drum

SACCADIC AND SEM TESTING
Procedure
1 Sit the patient facing you and ask them to fixate on a single target within their visual field.
2 Present a second target at a separate point within the field – this need not be in a specific position, as saccadic function is not dependent on position – and ask the patient to fix on the new target.
3 Repeat until you are satisfied that saccades are present or abnormal.
4 Carry out the testing for both horizontal and vertical saccades.
5 To test pursuit movements, slowly bring the same target across the visual field, initially horizontally, then vertically, and ask the patient to follow it whilst keeping their head still.
    ➤ Take care to present the target within the patient's visual field; this can be tested grossly before testing commences.
6 Present the optokinetic nystagmus drum to the patient, holding it either horizontally or vertically, and spin the drum slowly while observing the saccades.

DUCTION TESTING
Duction testing is undertaken to:
- identify muscle underaction, overaction or restriction
- establish binocular function.

The context for these tests may be in acute pathology (e.g. CN VI palsy) or for surgical planning (e.g. prior to strabismus surgery). Ideally, a non-accommodative target such as a spot light or pin should be used, as this reduces the effect of accommodative convergence.

PROCEDURE
1 Observe the patient for signs of an abnormal head posture (AHP) – in this situation, the head is held eccentrically, with the eyes aligned towards the target.
2 It is often a sign of ocular misalignment, although may be physiological or due to a non-ocular pathology; for example, torticollis. If possible, you should correct any AHP before proceeding.
3 Test versions first, then repeat the procedure for ductions by covering each eye in turn
4 Present the non-accommodative target (such as a bright light) to the patient in the primary position and move this to each of the six cardinal positions. The pattern of testing may be either an 'H' or a star (Union Jack).
5 Test the muscles in their position of primary action. Elevation and depression in the midline is the result of the action of a number of muscles – testing in vertical midline does not demonstrate single-muscle action. However, 'A'- and 'V'-pattern deviations are revealed by testing in this position, so this should be undertaken.
6 Observe and record comitancy and incomitancy.

Pearls

▶ Isolate the muscles to be tested:
  — vertical recti should be tested in abduction
  — obliques are tested in adduction – this reduces their torsional action.
▶ An apparent overaction of an antagonist may be observed, as well as underaction of the yoked muscle (Hering's law), this may be seen as a long-term sequela of CN IV palsy.
▶ Ocular motility can be more formally assessed using the Lees or Hess screen, which produces the Hess chart. This device dissociates the eyes and allows for quantitative representation of under- and overactions.

RECORDING EYE MOVEMENTS

Use standardised notation to record the findings of your examination.

In the diagrammatic notation, each eye is represented by its muscle actions, with a point noted for each muscle's position of action. Under- and overactions may be recorded as curved arrows in the muscle's position or as numerical approximations of the action, where '0' is normal. Failures of ductions are recorded as a shaded area in the area of underaction. These are graded from 0 to –4 on a linear scale, where '0' represents full action and '–4' no action whatsoever. In cases of complete palsy, the action of the antagonist may pull the eye across the midline – this is graded –5.

Eye movements may be recorded more objectively using a Lees screen. The Lees screen dissociates the eyes and compares each muscle's extent of action with standard excursions. Using this device, an orthoptist can record a Hess chart, which provides readily interpretable maps and may help to differentiate between restrictive and paretic movement limitation.

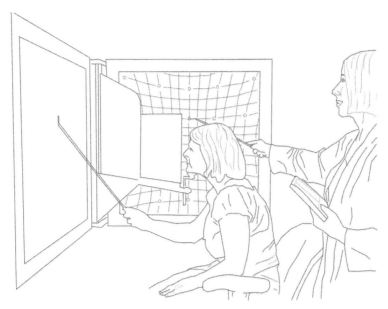

FIGURE CA7.2 Use of the Lees screen

AN APPROACH TO DIPLOPIA

Double vision a is vague symptom that frequently means very different things to the patient and the clinician. Therefore, it is important to have a structured approach to the investigation, diagnosis and management of double vision and diplopia.

The patient may describe symptoms such as blur, metamorphopsia, paracentral scotoma or refractive aberration as double vision. Clinicians define 'diplopia' as the perception of two images in place of a single fused image. Thus, the first step in the approach to a patient complaining of double vision is to take a careful and detailed history, eliciting exactly what it is that the patient is experiencing.

Monocular diplopia

Refractive aberrations may be described by patients as double vision or blur circles, particularly around points of light. These are perceived binocularly but remain when one eye is covered, thus revealing them to be monocular. They are common in patients with cataract; in particular, nuclear and posterior subcapsular types. Comatic aberration is common in patients with corneal ectasia and it may change over time. Other types of aberration may be described as double vision; particularly, the dysphotoptic symptoms caused by lens pits following yttrium aluminium garnet (YAG) capsulotomy. Peripheral iridotomies causing polycoria may result in monocular diplopia or dysphotopsia.

It is therefore important to establish if the symptom is present only when both eyes are open and fixing, or when one eye is covered. Monocular diplopia is always caused by refractive aberration, which is usually intraocular. First-time high plus prescriptions may produce jack-in-the-box edge effects that may be described by the patient as double vision. These are resolved by adaptation to the spectacles or by substituting contact lenses. Only double vision that is present with both eyes open is binocular; this is due to ocular misalignment – which may equally be termed a failure of comitance.

Binocular diplopia

Variations in comitancy of the eyes in various positions of gaze give variable diplopic symptoms. The images may be horizontally, vertically or obliquely distracted from each other – this relationship may change in various positions of gaze.

Horizontal and vertical diplopia may be classified as crossed or uncrossed, depending on the alignment of the visual axes. This can be readily established by asking the patient to fixate on a target within the diplopic field then repeatedly cover and uncover one eye. The patient should then be asked which image disappears (right or left in horizontal diplopia; top or bottom in vertical diplopia). If the image on the same side as the covered eye disappears, this is described as 'uncrossed' and indicates crossed, or esodeviated, eyes ('uncrossed' diplopia – crossed eyes; 'crossed' diplopia – uncrossed eyes). In the case of vertical diplopia, the upper image belongs to the lower eye – although this may not be the pathologically deviating eye (a right hypotropia might equally be described as a left hypertropia).

Before undertaking any examination, it is important to take a clinical history. Is the diplopia horizontally separated, vertically separated, or both, or is there an element of tilting? Is it worse when reading? This information will tell you which muscles may be involved.

Procedure

Vertical diplopia is best approached systematically using the Parks three-step test.
1 Identify the higher eye and the lower eye by occluding one eye and asking the patient, 'Which image disappears?'
   ➤ The higher image will disappear when the hypotropic eye is occluded.
   ➤ The lower image will disappear when the hypertropic eye is occluded.
   ➤ Corneal light reflexes may also be used to identify the deviating eye.
   ➤ Once the deviating eye is identified, there can be only four possible responsible muscles (the depressors of the hypertropic eye or the elevators of the hypotropic eye).
2 Identify if the responsible muscle is a vertical rectus or an oblique
   ➤ Test the recti in abduction and obliques in adduction.
   ➤ Is the diplopia present in abduction or adduction?

> After this stage, there can only be two possible responsible muscles (recti if diplopia is worse in abduction; obliques if diplopia is worse in abduction).
3 Identify the single responsible muscle.
> In the diplopic lateral position of gaze, ask the patient to look up and down.
> If the diplopia is greatest in elevation, the weak muscle must be the elevator of the hypotropic eye; if the diplopia is greater in depression, it is the depressor of the hypertropic eye.

SO palsy (CN IV palsy) characteristically causes elevation in adduction on the affected side and may be identified or confirmed with the Bielschowsky's head-tilt test. The SO (together with the SR) is an intorter – the antagonists are the inferior oblique and inferior rectus. A patient with an SO palsy may present with an AHP, with their head tilted away from the affected side.
1 Correct the AHP (after confirming the absence of co-morbidities which might preclude manipulation of the cervical spine)
2 The patient should fix a target in the primary position
3 Tilt the head towards the affected side
4 Observe for elevation of the eye on the affected side

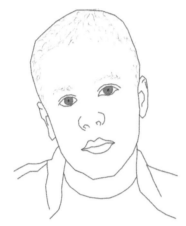

FIGURE CA7.3A A child with unilateral (in this case, left) SO underaction may demonstrate an AHP

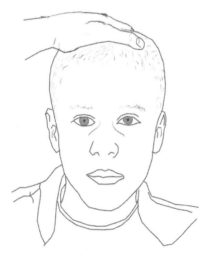

FIGURE CA7.3B Correct the AHP prior to testing

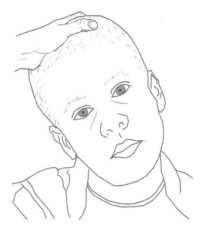

FIGURE CA7.3C Tilt the patient's head away from the affected side; the eyes remain aligned

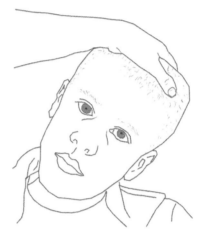

FIGURE CA7.3D Tilt the head towards the affected side. In the absence of SO function, the action of its synergist, the SR, is evident as the eye elevates

CODE: CA7
TARGET YEAR: 2

BASIC PRINCIPLES

Alignment of the eyes is a prerequisite for binocular single vision (BSV). Thus, it follows that failure of alignment denies the visual system the opportunity to develop or maintain complete BSV and stereopsis. The alignment need not be foveal, as anomalous retinal correspondence may coexist with some BSV, although the field of BSV may be reduced in these individuals. Nevertheless, high-quality vision (with foveal fixation), with good alignment of both eyes, provides the greatest stimulus for BSV and is likely to result in the largest field of BSV possible. Therefore, there are strong drivers to maintain eye alignment. When this breaks down, strabismus is present.

The physiological mechanisms for the maintenance of ocular alignment require approximately equal visual input from both eyes, an intact visual pathway, normal brainstem function and intact efferent pathways through the CN nuclei and fascicular pathways as well as, ultimately, normal extraocular muscle function. Discrepancies in any of these may result in strabismus, and the correct source must be identified in order to manage these cases adequately.

There are two types of strabismic deviation:

1 phorias: 'latent' deviations, which are only seen when fusion is disrupted or the eyes are dissociated
2 tropias: 'manifest' deviations, which are apparent without the removal of fusional control.

The direction of the deviation is prefixed to this classification; thus, an 'exophoria' describes an eye that becomes divergent only when dissociated (e.g. under cover, or at the Lees screen), while an 'esotropia' is seen when one eye remains convergent while both eyes are open.

CLINICAL APPLICATION

In clinical terms, the most straightforward way to remove fusional mechanisms is to occlude the eye. This denies bilateral visual stimuli and allows the covered eye to relax into its physiologically null position. Thus, cover testing is the basis of the investigation of strabismus.

Pearls

▸ Undertake the cover and uncover test on each eye in turn. Where a phoria is found, its maximal angle can be revealed by the alternate cover test. This maximally dissociates the eyes and reveals the true extent of a phoria.

▸ Cover testing should be undertaken both for near and distance, with and without spectacle correction. In this way, various patterns of deviation, such as accommodative esodeviations and simulated distance exodeviations, may be diagnosed. The targets should be accommodative to stimulate real-world deviation.

EQUIPMENT LIST:

● Near and distance targets
● Occluder

- Prism bar or free prisms
- Light source – e.g. a direct ophthalmoscope

PROCEDURE

> ### Cover testing – general points
> Perform cover testing both with and without appropriate refractive correction, and with both a distance and a near fixation target (which should be held by the patient at arm's length).
> 1 Observe the patient for the presence of AHP (this should be corrected if present) and for manifest strabismus.
> 2 Taking care not to occlude the visual axis with your body, occlude the eyes from above, resting the heel of your hand on the patient's forehead, and swinging the occluder from eye to eye from this position.

Detecting a manifest deviation

The **cover test** is used to demonstrate the presence of a manifest deviation.
1 To find a manifest deviation, observe the corneal reflex from a bright spot illumination at 1 m – the reflex should be roughly central and equal; a unilaterally non-central reflex suggests a deviating eye (Hirschberg test).
2 If a manifest deviation is seen, the fixating eye should be covered first.
3 Leave the cover in place for 2–3 seconds – the deviating eye should be observed moving to take up fixation.

Detecting a latent deviation

The **uncover test** demonstrates latent (-phoric) strabismus.
  Undertake a cover test as above then uncover the eye and look for a refixation saccade (the covered, therefore, non-fixing, eye will deviate if a phoria is present).

Alternate cover test

The **alternate cover test** is used to measure manifest (tropic) and latent (phoric) deviation and is a continuation of the cover test.
1 Cover first the fixing eye then its fellow, sequentially.
2 Never allow binocular vision during alternate cover testing, but leave the cover over one eye for a second or two, then cover its fellow again.
  ➤ The angle of the phoria will often increase rapidly during alternate testing.
3 Assess control of the phoria after alternate cover testing by removing the occluder and watching for control.

Prism cover test

The **prism cover test** allows for quantitative assessment and documentation of the angle of deviation.
1 Perform a cover test (*see* above) to identify the side and type of deviation, then make an estimation of the size of the deviation.
2 Occlude the deviating eye and put a prism of approximately appropriate power in front of the occluder with its *apex towards the direction of the deviation*.
3 Remove the occluder and observe the movement of the eye.
4 Fine-tune the prism strength until no movement is seen on uncovering the eye.
5 Check alignment under the prism using the corneal light reflex, which should be in the same position on each eye when they are aligned (Krimsky test).

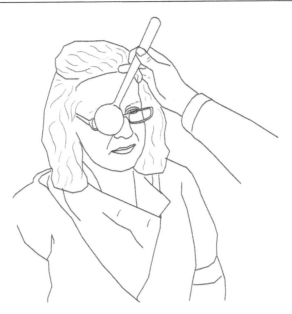

FIGURE CA7.4 Cover test

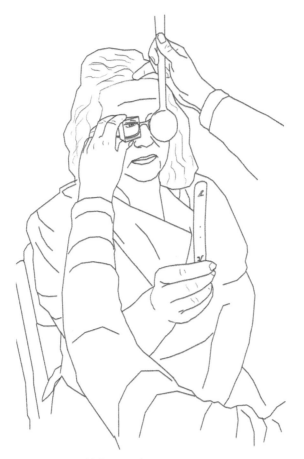

FIGURE CA7.5 Prism cover test with loose prism

Applanation tonometry

CODE: CA8
TARGET YEAR: 1

BACKGROUND
Assessment of the pressure inside a fluid-filled sphere may be made by measuring the force required to flatten a part of its surface, when the thickness and rigidity of the surface is known. This is the basis of applanation tonometry, in which the plane anterior surface of a split prism of known diameter is used to flatten the surface of the cornea.

The Imbert–Fick principle is the mathematical basis for the technique of applanation tonometry and makes several assumptions about the cornea that are known to be false. The cornea is assumed to be spherical, infinitely thin and have no rigidity or capacity to stretch; in practice, none of these assumptions is true. The principle, however, remains acceptable as a gold-standard technique and will continue to do so until corneal biomechanics are fully understood and characterised.

CLINICAL APPLICATION
A split prism with a radius of 3.06 mm is placed against the anaesthetised cornea. The clinician judges the point of corneal flattening by aligning the mires created by the tear meniscus (hence the need for a split prism) and reads the pressure from the gauge.

The principle is the same whether the process is undertaken at the slit lamp (Goldmann tonometer) or with a portable system (Perkins tonometer).

EQUIPMENT LIST
- Slit-lamp biomicroscope with Goldmann tonometer *or* Perkins applanation tonometer
- Goldmann tonometer prism
- Combined 0.5% fluorescein and topical anaesthetic drop *or* Fluorets® strip and topical anaesthetic drop

PROCEDURE
Slit-lamp biomicroscope with Goldmann tonometer
1 Instil dye and anaesthetic into the inferior conjunctival fornix.
2 Ensure the patient's position at the slit lamp is correct.
3 Align an appropriately disinfected tonometer prism in the mount.
  ➤ Align the white marking line on the prism with the white line on the mount.
  ➤ Use the red marker on the prism when high corneal astigmatism is present (*see* 'Pearls', p. 23).
4 Select low magnification power with bright illumination through the cobalt blue filter.
5 Swing the illumination arm to between 45 and 90 degrees on the same side as the eye being examined.
6 Dial the tonometer to a value close to the expected pressure.
7 Retract the eyelids.
8 Advance the carriage forwards until the tonometer touches the cornea and a blue reflex can be observed.
9 Observe the fluorescent mires through a single eyepiece.
10 Dial the tonometer gauge until the inside edges of the mires just touch.

Perkins tonometer

If using a Perkins tonometer, the procedure is the same as that for the slit lamp and Goldmann tonometer, except that the instrument is rested on the patient's forehead using the pad.

Pearls

- Take care to avoid putting pressure on the globe with your fingers as you retract the lids.
  - Support the upper lid margin on the orbital rim and the inferior lid on the superior maxilla.
- If there is significant pulsation of the reflex, take the reading at the midpoint of the wavelength.
- This tonometry technique is based on corneal resistance to being deformed by the tonometer.
  - This may be affected by corneal thickness and rigidity. Therefore, the reading is prone to error in anatomically unusual corneas; for example, those:
    - » that are excessively thick or thin
    - » following refractive surgery
    - » following corneal collagen cross-linking therapy.
- High corneal astigmatism may cause error in the mire configuration. In these cases, the red line on the mount should be used and the steep axis aligned with this mark using the gauge on the prism.

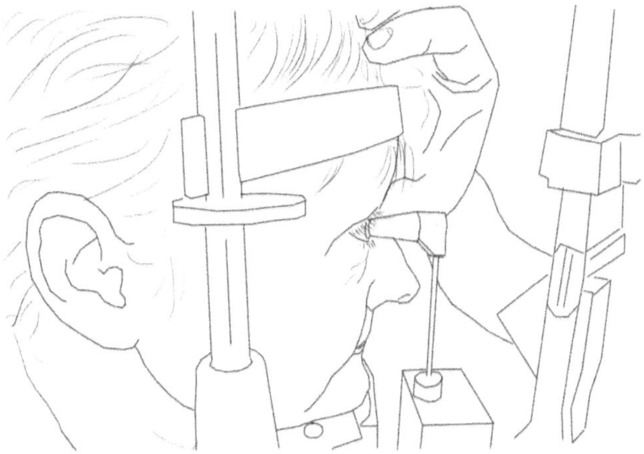

FIGURE CA8.1 Take care not to apply digital pressure to the globe during applanation tonometry

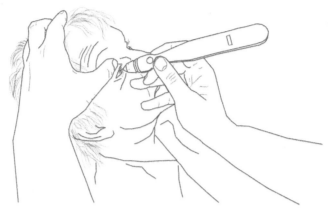

FIGURE CA8.2 The Tono-Pen® (Reichert, USA) provides accurate intraocular-pressure measurement in patients who are unable to position on the slit lamp. Rebound tonometers may also be used in this context

Pearl

▶ Keep the Tono-Pen® perpendicular to the cornea and allow a blink in between recording with light taps on the centre of the cornea after instilling anaesthetic drops.

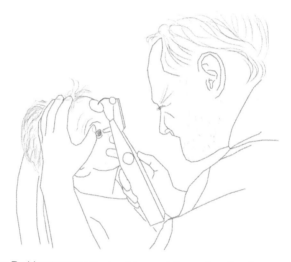

FIGURE CA8.3 The Perkins tonometer provides mobile applanation tonometry

Slit lamp

CODE: CA9
TARGET YEAR: 1

BACKGROUND

The slit lamp is the primary instrument of investigation for the Ophthalmologist, and competent use of this piece of equipment will allow thorough and extensive examination of the globe and adnexal structures.

The slit lamp is composed of two parts, a biomicroscope of fixed focal length and an illumination column. They are both fixed around a common axis that is coincident with their focal points, but each can be rotated about this point independently. Attached to the assembly is the patient's chin rest and forehead band, which ensures the head is kept still. The chin rest can be adjusted up and down with a worm screw, which is found on the side assembly. The lateral canthal angle should be aligned with the mark on the vertical bar. The patient is encouraged to rest comfortably with their chin on the rest and forehead against the band.

Control of the biomicroscope is via the joystick and the illumination arm. Coarse movements are made by moving the entire assembly forwards and backwards; finer control for focusing and examination is via smaller movements of the joystick. Rotation of the joystick clockwise will move both observation and illumination assemblies down; anticlockwise rotation will move the assembly up. The examiner should set their own inter-pupillary distance and eyepiece focus so as to obtain a crisp single image through the binocular biomicroscope.

The orientation of illumination, and the breadth and length of the beam as well as filters, are controlled on the illumination arm.

The illumination and observation arms may be decoupled in order to undertake various examination techniques (see below). The illumination may be rotated around the X-axis to improve perception of depth.

The filters available vary from model to model, but most slit lamps have the following filters:

- cobalt blue:
  - used for excitation of dilute fluorescein dye – assessment of corneal/conjunctival epithelial injury, Goldmann tonometry
  - may also be used to demonstrate autofluorescence.
- red-free:
  - used to demonstrate haemorrhage.
- polarising:
  - halves the illumination and is used for visualising anterior-chamber cells.
- infrared:
  - used to prevent thermal injury to the retina.

SLIT-LAMP TECHNIQUES

The coincident but unaligned viewing and illumination components of the slit lamp allow for various examination and illumination techniques. A knowledge of and skill in these techniques allow the examiner to take advantage of the various optical properties of the eye to find and identify pathology. There are seven techniques for the examination of the adnexa and anterior segment; the trainee Ophthalmologist should be familiar with how and when to use each of them.

1 Diffuse illumination:
  ➤ the anterior structures are illuminated with a wide, filtered beam; the illumination arm may be coaxial or within 45 degrees of that position
  ➤ the technique involves a lid and corneal surface examination, as well as examination of the properties of the tear film when used with fluorescein.

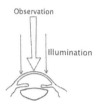

FIGURE CA9.1 Diffuse illumination

2 Oblique illumination:
  ➤ a bright, narrow, white slit beam is directed at the corneal surface from an oblique position. The microscope may be moved to maximise the angle between the illumination and viewing axes
  ➤ the anterior and posterior curvature of the cornea are assessed.

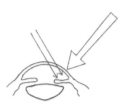

FIGURE CA9.2 Oblique illumination

3 Direct illumination:
  ➤ the illuminating arm and the biomicroscope are held around 45 degrees from each other, and the light is focused on the area of interest
  ➤ use direct illumination to examine conjunctival, lid and iris lesions.

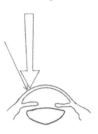

FIGURE CA9.3 Direct illumination

4 Retroillumination:
  ➤ the illumination and observing arms are arranged in a coaxial configuration. Light is directed through the pupil and is reflected by the retina (red reflex)
  ➤ the technique assesses posterior capsular opacification, iris transillumination defects and the patency of peripheral iridotomies.

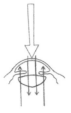

FIGURE CA9.4 Retroillumination

5 Sclerotic scatter:
   ➤ the illumination and observing arms are decoupled, and the sclera just posterior
     to the limbus is brightly illuminated, while the corneal stroma is observed.
     Light transmitted via the limbus undergoes total internal reflection through the
     stroma, highlighting pathology that may not be evident with other techniques
   ➤ use sclerotic scatter to examine stromal scars and dystrophies.

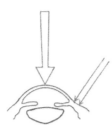

FIGURE CA9.5 Sclerotic scatter

6 Indirect illumination:
   ➤ use a bright, narrow illumination directed adjacent to corneal lesions
   ➤ similar to sclerotic scatter, this technique demonstrates stromal opacities, while
     allowing for more extensive assessment of the cornea and anterior segment.

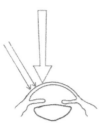

FIGURE CA9.6 Indirect illumination

7 Specular illumination:
   ➤ a very bright, narrow beam is used, with the viewing arm arranged either side of
     perpendicular at equal angles
   ➤ the technique examines the endothelial cells.

FIGURE CA9.7 Specular illumination

Fundus examination: direct ophthalmoscopy

CODE: CA10
TARGET YEAR: 2
AIM: to examine the macula and optic-nerve head for the identification of pathology.

EQUIPMENT LIST
- Mydriatic agent
- Fluorescein dye (1%–2%)
- Direct ophthalmoscope

PROCEDURE
1 Complete an examination of the pupil (*see* CA6, p. 10).
2 Instil the mydriatic agent.
3 Dial your own refractive correction into the lens rack.

Examination of the red reflex
1 From an arm's length, swing a bright white illuminating beam across the eye with a dilated pupil.
 ➤ The red reflex should glow brightly and be of broadly uniform intensity and colour.

Examination of the cornea
1 Add +10 dioptres (D) of refracting power on the lens rack.
2 Examine the cornea using retroillumination against the red reflex.
3 Instil fluorescein dye and use the blue filter to identify areas of epithelial loss.

Examination of the lens
1 Reduce power until the cornea comes into focus.
2 Advance to within 5 cm of the cornea.
3 Visualise lens opacities under either direct illumination or retroillumination.

Examination of the posterior segment
1 Reduce the refractive power of the instrument to the sum of the examiner's and the subject's refractive error.
2 Remain at least 5 cm from the corneal surface.
3 Visualise retinal features under direct illumination.
4 Adjust the focus by either moving the instrument in an anteroposterior direction, or changing the refractive power.

Pearls
▶ The direct ophthalmoscope provides a virtual, erect image.
▶ Corneal features, including grafts, pannus, ectasia and pigment deposition, are all visible with the direct ophthalmoscope.
▶ The magnification is high and the field of view is very small, so do not expect to see an extensive vista of the posterior segment.
▶ The optic disc is nasal to the macula, therefore can be visualised by approaching the patient from their lateral side.
▶ Find a retinal vessel bifurcation then follow it back to the disc.
▶ Retinal veins are thicker and a deeper red compared with the arteries.
▶ Small haemorrhages are more easily seen under red-free (green) illumination.

SKILL Fundus examination: slit-lamp indirect ophthalmoscopy

CODE: CA10
TARGET YEAR: 2
AIM: to examine the central and peripheral retina for the identification of pathology at the slit lamp.

EQUIPMENT LIST
- Mydriatic agent
- Slit-lamp biomicroscope
- Condensing lens (60–90 D)

PROCEDURE
1 Complete an examination of the pupil (*see* CA6, p. 10).
2 Instil the mydriatic.
3 Ensure the illumination arm and microscope are coaxial.
4 The illumination should be low and the diffusing filter selected.
5 Start with the carriage at its most rearward point.
6 Identify the red reflex.
7 Place the condensing lens around 3 cm in front of the cornea, supporting your hand on the head band of the slit lamp.
8 Advance the carriage towards the red reflex until the retinal image comes into focus.
9 If you lose the image, move the carriage backwards and once again obtain the red reflex through the condensing lens.
10 Examine the macula and disc before moving to the peripheral retina.

Pearls
▶ The slit-lamp indirect examination technique provides a real, inverted image.
▶ Different condensing lenses provide varying fields of view and, consequently, magnification:
— the 90 D lens provides a wide field of view, through a small pupil
— the 78 D lens provides reasonable views to the equator and of the disc
— the 66 D lens provides highly magnified views of the macula and disc
— specialist wide-angle and high-magnification lenses exist.
▶ Navigate the retina by moving both the lens and the slit lamp, and also by asking the patient to look towards each quadrant in turn.
▶ Notation should be erect and laterally correct – you must either become accustomed to reconfiguring the image in your mind before drawing it or, alternatively, turn the page upside down and record findings as they appear.

CODE: CA10

TARGET YEARS: 4–7

AIM: to use the binocular indirect ophthalmoscope to examine the central and peripheral retina.

EQUIPMENT LIST

- Examination couch or adjustable chair
- Binocular indirect ophthalmoscope
- Condensing lenses:
  - ➤ 20 D
  - ➤ 28 D
  - ➤ pan-retinal
- Mydriatic agent and topical anaesthesia
- Scleral indenter

PROCEDURE

Indirect ophthalmoscopy is best undertaken with the patient supine. A flat examination couch, with good access to each side of the head, is preferable, although this is frequently impractical; at the very least, the patient should be reclined.

1. Dilate the patient's pupils.
2. Position the patient and explain the procedure.
3. Set the ophthalmoscope to a dim illumination with a medium-sized spot.
4. Adjust the fit of the headband so that the instrument is secure.
5. Adjust the position of each eyepiece in turn, so that it is possible to fuse the illumination spot on a hand held at 33 cm.
6. Hold the lens with thumb and forefinger, with the marking ring (usually a silver ring on one side of the lens rim) facing the patient.
7. Rest the heel of your hand on the patient's forehead, stabilising the lens in front of the eye.
8. Standing around an arm's length away, illuminate the lens and adjust the position of your head and the lens until an image is formed.
9. Move around the patient and direct their gaze to examine the peripheral retina.
10. If indentation is required, instil further topical anaesthesia.
11. Hold the scleral indenting thimble between the thumb and forefinger.
12. Place the tip of the indenter within the conjunctival fornix or over the lid in the skin crease (direct scleral indentation is very uncomfortable for the patient).
13. Rotate the shaft of the indenter around the tip, applying gentle pressure on the wall of the globe while examining the same area of retina.
14. To dynamically examine the vitreous base and peripheral breaks, gently move the tip in an anteroposterior (AP) direction.

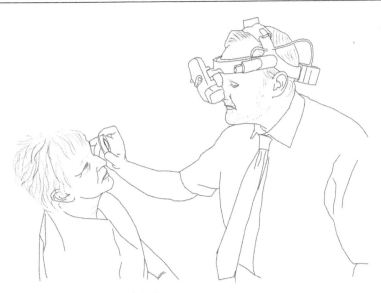

FIGURE CA10 Binocular indirect ophthalmoscopy

Patient investigation

Corneal shape, structure and thickness

CODE: PI2
TARGET YEAR OF ACHIEVEMENT: 2

BACKGROUND

The shape and clarity of the cornea, the chief refracting structure of the eye, are paramount to ensuring the effective transmission of light to the neurosensory retina. The ability of the cornea to transmit light is affected by its microstructure, and its ability to focus light onto the retina is affected by its shape and surface quality. Modern imaging techniques are available to measure these properties and help the clinician make diagnoses and plan management. Basic examinations include corneal topography, corneal-thickness measurement and corneal biomicroscopy. The trainee should have a firm grasp of the techniques, their execution and interpretation.

CORNEAL TOPOGRAPHY

At the most basic level, the evaluation of gross topographical features of the corneal surface may be made at the slit lamp. A bright, unfiltered beam with a narrow, oblique slit and high magnification passed laterally over the cornea will afford the examiner an impression of the anterior and posterior curvatures and thicknesses. Corneal ectasia may be relatively easy to identify, especially when other signs such as Vogt's striae or Fleischer rings are observed. The corneal structure may be examined in section by adjusting the position of the viewing system so that corneal form and cone location may be assessed. However, early ectasia and forme fruste keratoconus may only be identifiable with topographic mapping.

The first topographic instruments were simple optical devices (Placido's rings and discs), which were handheld and allowed direct observation of the anterior curvature, although quantitative measurements were challenging or impossible. Modern videokeratoscopy is largely based on the same principles. A pattern of concentric rings is projected onto the cornea, and their reflection is acquired by a digital camera; the images are then analysed for compression of the rings relating to corneal steepening. The development of slit imaging technologies has allowed the Ophthalmologist to view corneal *tomography*, which incorporates an analysis of the posterior as well as the anterior surfaces of the cornea. The major advantage of this is the ability to view corneal thickness across the cornea, where decentration of the minimum corneal thickness from the central point is highly indicative of ectatic disease. Best-fit reference shapes generated for each surface show 'elevation' differences from expected norms, and such protrusion of shape is useful in monitoring and diagnosis.

Orbscan™ (Bausch and Lomb, USA) uses a combination of Placido-based anterior topography, and slit-scanning techniques for posterior-curve and corneal-thickness evaluation. Slit-scan imaging as used in the Orbscan system is essentially an automated version of the slit-lamp examination. Forty very narrow slits are centred on the corneal apex then rotated. The high-resolution video camera detects these images and processes data from 240 data points per slit.

The Pentacam™ (Oculus, Germany) system is based on the Scheimpflug principle, which states that an optical system with a fixed depth of focus will produce crisp images of its subject only if that subject is uniplanar, parallel with the lens and within the area of focus; if the plane of the subject is not coincident with the lens, parts of it will be out of focus (in front and behind the focal point). To overcome this, the lens must be rotated about the focal point, until it and the subject's plane are coincident. In the case of a curved surface, such as the cornea, this requires constant readjustment of the lens position. By measuring the excursion of the lens as it finds the focused image, the Pentacam can map the curvature of the corneal surface. Scheimpflug cameras obtain very high-resolution images of curved surfaces, and, when used in conjunction with ultrasound biomicroscopy (UBM), render enormously detailed images of anterior-segment structures.

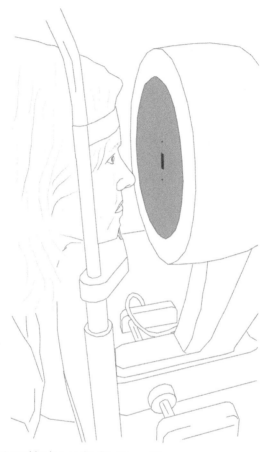

FIGURE PI2.1 Correct positioning at the Pentacam™

With all systems, the user is given colour-coded maps of the cornea. The maps may relate to various parameters including anterior or posterior curvature or refractive power, corneal thickness or deviation from standard models. The colours used are not standard, and the scale may be altered by the user – it is therefore important to check the calibration before reading a scan.

The use of handheld optical systems is now outmoded in modern practice. The peculiarities of each automated system are their own, but, in general the measurements are acquired automatically. Good tear film and minimal eye movements are essential for reliable corneal topography. The user must ensure adequate patient positioning on the chin rest, with proper vertical alignment. Each system uses its own type of focusing cue, but usually the user must focus the camera on the anterior cornea centrally – automatic image capture and pupil tracking then take over to complete acquisition of the image.

Alongside topographic mapping, the systems provide quantitative data for the user. Generally, the examiner is interested in the curvature (for diagnosis) and the refractive power of the cornea (for management planning). Thus, the most useful data provided are the 'simulated Ks', which give measurements of corneal curvature in the central 3 mm, and the dioptric power maps.

Other data fields that may be available include the index of asphericity (used in the planning of laser correction of refractive error), indices related to corneal surface regularity (surface regularity index) and corneal clarity (corneal uniformity index and predicted corneal acuity) – these parameters are primarily designed for use in laser-refractive correction and, as such, the detailed examination of these functions is beyond the scope of this text.

The skill in corneal topography comes in identifying the patterns demonstrated and their clinical implications (*see* Figure PI2.2, colour plate).

CORNEAL CONFOCAL MICROSCOPY AND SPECULAR MICROSCOPY

The simplest way to examine the cornea is with careful and methodical use of the slit lamp. However, increasingly, technological advances are allowing for high-quality imaging at higher magnifications than are practical at the slit lamp.

The very properties of the cornea that make it ideal for the transmission of light also confound the efforts of traditional photographic techniques. There is very little scatter and diffraction within the healthy cornea, making capturing reflected light difficult. Further, patient movement and microsaccades of the eye do not permit very high-magnification examination at the slit lamp.

Two techniques have evolved to overcome these problems, and both have their place in the cornea clinic.

Confocal microscopy

This technique, derived from very-high-magnification techniques used in applied cellular biology, allows high-resolution scanning of coronal sections of the cornea. The confocal microscope employs a beam splitter and pinholes to significantly reduce scatter and ensure a consistent depth of field. The corneal surface is scanned using multiple pinhole-filtered beams, and the image is reconstructed. Confocal microscopy is particularly useful for the quantitative analysis of endothelial-cell populations in endothelial dystrophies and for the in vivo diagnosis of atypical keratitis. It is also of use for the planning of laser-refractive surgery.

Automated specular microscopy

Examination of the corneal endothelium at the slit lamp using specular illumination demonstrates the principles of specular microscopy. As only light reflected towards the viewing system is perceived by the viewer and the angle of reflectance is equal to the angle of incidence, the user must manipulate the angle of incidence so that reflected light arrives within their percept. Reflectance occurs at the interface of surfaces of differing refractive indices; the corneal endothelium has evolved with a refractive index very close to that of water (aqueous), consequently, only around 0.02% of incident light is reflected from this interface. Image quality and resolution is rapidly degraded by scatter at the interfaces, and, when the amount of light reflected is proportionally so low, this results in very poor image resolution (as seen at the slit lamp). Automated specular microscopes overcome this problem by excluding all light that is not directly reflected (excluding scattered light) to the viewing system. This produces higher resolution imaging of cellular interfaces and quantitative analysis of sheets of cells – for example, the corneal endothelium (normal cell density reduces from 3400 cells/mm^2 at age 15 years to 2300 cells/mm^2 at age 85 years).

From the examiner's point of view, the process of acquiring these images is largely automated. The patient should be positioned appropriately at the camera, and the image roughly aligned. The camera's autofocus and tracking control will then take over.

CORNEAL PACHYMETRY

The healthy cornea has a central thickness of around 550 nm and peripherally, near the limbus, of up to 850 nm. An accurate assessment of the thickness of the cornea aids in the diagnosis of many corneal diseases as well as informing the results of Goldmann tonometry in the glaucoma clinic.

There are several techniques for the measurement of corneal thickness. The trainee should be aware of these; however, the most commonly used is ultrasound pachymetry. Historically, the most frequently used were optical systems, and these still exist. As more modern ophthalmic imaging techniques proliferate, the task of pachymetry may fall to optical coherence tomography (OCT), Scheimpflug cameras, confocal microscopy or corneal waveform (a variation of ultrasonic techniques).

Ultrasound pachymetry

A pencil-sized A-scan ultrasound probe is placed onto the anaesthetised cornea without coupling fluid. Multiple single waves are emitted from the probe, and the reflectance from the endothelium–aqueous interface is received. The probe averages the results from these multiple echoes and provides a value for corneal thickness with a confidence interval.

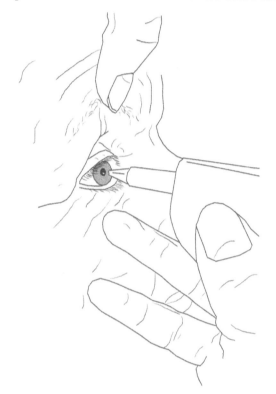

FIGURE PI2.3 A-scan pachymetry

This test is easy and quick to perform and is suitable for patients who are unable to position at the slit lamp. Set up of the handheld unit is simple, and it is automatically calibrated so that there is a high degree of repeatability in its examinations.

Optical pachymetry

'Optical pachymeters' are low-coherence reflectomers that measure the distance between reflections from the tear film and endothelium–aqueous interface. These systems may be added to a slit lamp or exist as purpose-built units, often integrating non-contact tonometric devices. They are non-contact systems and can be as accurate as ultrasound-based systems. However, accuracy is dependent on tear film, corneal clarity and the patient's ability to position themselves onto the machine's chin rest.

Ocular angiography

CODE: PI4
TARGET YEAR OF ACHIEVEMENT: 2
AIM: to be able to interpret fundus fluorescein angiograms and use the determined information to diagnose and devise treatment plans.

BACKGROUND

Fundus fluorescein angiography (FFA) is a standard investigative procedure in the medical retina clinic. It is used extensively in the diagnosis, monitoring and treatment planning of diabetic eye disease, choroidal neovascular disease, retinal vascular disease, neoplastic disease, and retinal and macular dystrophies. The advent of digital photographic techniques has further increased the power of this form of investigation, with modern software allowing the clinician to overlay information from colour photographs, FFA, OCT, scanning laser ophthalmoscopy (SLO) and stereo photography to more fully understand the pathological processes occurring in an eye.

When injected intravenously, fluorescein dye ($C_{20}H_{12}O_5$) is adsorbed by albumin and erythrocyte cell membranes – it does not diffuse into the cells. In blood, its light absorption peaks at 465 nm (blue) and its emission at 525 nm. It is this property which allows us to use the dye to demonstrate the pattern of fluid and blood movements within the vascular compartments of the retina (and to a lesser extent the choroid).

> **Pearl**
> ▶ The nomenclature associated with the reporting of FFA concerns the fluorescence pattern of dye penetration and can be divided into those patterns which demonstrate hyperfluorescence and those which demonstrate hypofluorescence. 'Hyperfluorescence' patterns are window defects, leakage, staining and abnormal vessels. 'Hypofluorescences' are described as masking and filling defects (or 'dropouts').

It is important to establish a routine system for reporting on a fundus fluorescein angiogram, just as a radiologist or chest physician interrogates a chest X-ray. Thus, it is good practice (particularly in teaching and examinations) to start by commenting on the type of examination and laterality and to identify the patient (e.g. 'This is a fundus fluorescein angiogram of the right eye of Mrs Smith'). Detailed explanation of the potential findings in a fundus fluorescein angiogram follow, and the 'report' should include commentary on them, ending with a suggested diagnosis and justification for this.

A set of FFA images will typically start with colour and red-free images of the fundus (taken prior to the injection of dye). Subsequent images represent various stages of dye penetration through the vascular cycle. These are divided into five distinct phases, and these should be referred to in the report, as the fluorescence patterns alter with them. The phases are:
1 choroidal – initial blush of fluorescence within choroidal vessels
2 arterial – retinal arteries are full, with no fluorescence in veins
3 arteriovenous – laminar flow of dye within veins, with fluorescing capillaries
4 venous – retinal veins full
5 late – all vessels fluoresce, commonly with some staining at disc

A representative image from each of these phases should be chosen for closer inspection,

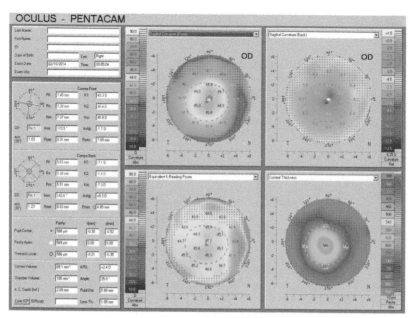

FIGURE PI2.2 Pentacam™ maps demonstrating keratoconus. Anterior and posterior elevation maps, corneal-thickness and keratometric power-deviation maps are displayed. Keratometric indices are displayed alongside

and a systematic approach to each of these images undertaken. FFA is a dynamic investigation; that is, the pattern of findings may change over the course of the test. Thus, it is impossible to adequately report on an FFA investigation based on a single frame. In particular, the discrimination in hyperfluorescence caused by staining or leakage is critical and can only be appreciated with a complete run of images.

FFA is considered an investigative procedure rather than an examination, and should not be interpreted in isolation from either a clinical assessment or colour photograph of the fundus.

PATTERNS OF HYPERFLUORESCENCE

'Hyperfluorescence' indicates apparent increased concentrations of dye within the tissue. This may be due to extravasation of dye into the tissues compared with into the adjacent areas, staining of the tissue with dye, increased visibility of the dye in deeper layers due to deficiency in overlying retinal pigment (window defect) or vascular abnormality.

PATTERNS OF HYPOFLUORESCENCE

Areas of the retina or vessels that do not fluoresce as brightly as adjacent tissue of the same type are said to be 'hypofluorescent'. These areas may be physiological (foveal avascular zone [FAZ] 450–600 µm) or pathological. Pathological areas of hypofluorescence may be due to poor vascular filling or the masking of deeper structures. Vascular hypoperfusion is related to capillary non-perfusion (seen as wedges of hypofluorescence in the retinal capillary bed) or retinal vessel non-perfusion. The masking of the fluorescence of deeper layers by non-perfusing overlying structures is an important cause of hypofluorescence and is most commonly due to pre- or intraretinal haemorrhage. It is important to identify the level of the blood – pre-retinal masking defects obscure retinal vessels, while intraretinal haemorrhages do not.

Patterns of fluorescence
- **Hyperfluorescence**
  - Staining
  - Leakage
  - Window defect
- **Hypofluorescence**
  - Physiological
  - Non-perfusion (dropout)
  - Masking defect

In many cases, a fundus fluorescein angiogram will demonstrate evidence of both hyper- and hypofluorescence. This is particularly true of the multiple causes of retinal ischaemia, as reduced tissue perfusion, haemorrhage and neovascularisation, with or without leakage of fluid into the retina, may all occur within the same eye. Thus, it is important to apply a systematic approach to the reporting of a fundus fluorescein angiogram so that one neither becomes bogged down by the minutiae nor neglects those signs which are not initially noted.

Although more modern techniques such as OCT and SLO have been developed since the advent of FFA, it remains an immensely powerful diagnostic aid and is likely to continue to be used for many years.

CODE: PI5
TARGET YEAR OF ACHIEVEMENT: 2
AIM: to be able to carry out ultrasound of the globe and orbit and interpret the findings.

BACKGROUND

The use of B-scan ultrasound in ophthalmic practice remains an important skill to master, and new applications for high-resolution ultrasound imaging techniques, such as UBM, are being found in both research and clinical fields. Previously common techniques, including A-scan, A-scan biometry and Doppler ultrasound, are still occasionally used, so it is important to be versed in their application and interpretation.

Ocular ultrasound modalities

- A-scan (amplitude modulation): this is the simplest form of ultrasound and consists of a single transduced wave. The echoes are displayed on screen, and the distance from each echogenic surface may be measured. This technique is employed in A-scan biometry to calculate axial length (AL) and anterior-chamber depth when lenticular opacity precludes the use of optical systems. Most modern ultrasound machines display an overlaid A-scan on the B-scan image – the position of this within the B-mode array can be changed by the user.
- B-scan (brightness scanning): the most commonly employed form of ocular ultrasound in clinical practice. A two-dimensional band of transduced waves (10 MHz) returns an array of echoes, which are reconstructed on screen to form a two-dimensional image. B-scan is used in ophthalmic practice for the identification of posterior-segment pathology, both for measurement of lesions and dynamic examination.
- Ultrasound biomicroscopy: this is an ultrasonic technique, which uses a significantly higher frequency of B-mode ultrasound (50 MHz) to image the tissues of the anterior segment in great detail.
- Doppler ultrasound: this technique makes use of the Doppler effect to measure the flow of a liquid. Although commonly employed in the vascular clinic, its use in ophthalmic practice is limited to the identification of the temporal artery prior to biopsy.

B-SCAN SETTINGS

The user can vary a number of parameters to achieve the best results from a B-scan examination.

- Decibel gain: the user may increase the frequency of the ultrasonic wave produced by the unit in order to adjust the resolution. As the gain is increased, the signal-to-noise ratio (SNR) is reduced, a consequence of which is a reduction in the resolution of the image. High gain settings are usually used to examine the vitreous and vitreo-retinal interface. Detailed anatomical examination of the retina and disc requiring higher resolution is more successfully undertaken with lower gain settings – in particular, when delineating the extrascleral penetration of tumours, examining optic-disc drusen and looking for evidence of calcification in retinoblastoma. Low gain B-scan ultrasonography has now been superseded by OCT imaging for many of the instances in which the former may have been used in the past.
- Greyscale: the B-scan image is made up of a number of grey dots displayed on the screen in varying brightness. The range of greys displayed may be manipulated.

More detailed images are formed with a wide greyscale, at the expense of contrast between structures.

- Anterior shift: the probe's depth of focus is fixed and engineered to display the structures of the posterior segment most clearly. In order to increase the detail of posterior segment tissues the user may suppress the part of the image that shows the anterior structures. This feature is rarely used in practice.

EQUIPMENT LIST

- B-scan ultrasound unit with a 10 MHz probe
- Ultrasonic gel

PROCEDURE

When undertaking a B-scan, it is important to be aware of the orientation of the array, as this will determine which tissues are examined. There is an orientation marker on the tip of the probe that corresponds to the axis of the array. By rotating the probe along its long axis, the examiner may manipulate the angle of incident sound waves, and, therefore, the structures examined.

Pearls
- The scanning beam should be centred over the area of interest.
- The probe should be directed so that waves are perpendicular to the structures of interest.
- Use the lowest gain settings possible whilst maintaining good resolution.

Screening of the retina is best undertaken in a systematic fashion, utilising all three sections. In all cases, the lids are closed, and the transducer is coupled to the skin using an aqueous gel:

1. axial section: the probe is placed over the central cornea, over the closed lid, and directed towards the optic-nerve head. This section provides views of the posterior pole, although image quality is compromised by the absorption of sound waves by the crystalline lens. Views of the peripheral retina are rather difficult using this section
2. transverse section: the probe is placed on the closed lid adjacent to the limbus, with the orientation marker perpendicular (by convention, nasally in the horizontal meridian and superiorly in the vertical). The probe should be smoothly shifted from limbus to fornix to examine the posterior pole and peripheral retina. Image quality is increased compared with axial sections, as the lens is excluded. Peripheral coverage is good, although it is easy to become disorientated. This section is particularly useful for measuring the posterior extent of lesions
3. longitudinal section: the probe is placed over the sclera with the marker facing the limbus with the lids closed. The patient is asked to direct their gaze away from the probe (towards the meridian to be examined). The longitudinal section demonstrates an AP section, which extends from the optic nerve to the ciliary body. It is useful for the demonstration of the AP extension of tumours and attachments to the optic-nerve head.

Ultrasound allows the user to measure lesions (quantitative examination) as well as demonstrate movement and anatomical connections (kinetic examination).

The importance of kinetic examination is underlined by the different behaviours of structures that may appear very similar on static examination. For example, distinguishing between choroidal effusion, retinal detachment and vitreous detachment would be difficult without dynamic (kinetic) examination, as each of these conditions appears as a membranous opacity with a similar configuration when viewed statically. However, choroidal effusions demonstrate no movement or after-movement on saccades; retinal detachments tend to demonstrate more movement with rapid inertial changes; and vitreous detachments are more mobile still, with slower inertial deceleration.

1   Position yourself, the patient, the machine and footswitch so that you can control the probe with your dominant hand, ensuring you have a clear view of the screen and easy access to the footswitch.

2   Ask the patient to close their eyes, and apply a generous volume of gel to the probe tip.

3   To acquire axial images, with the patient's eyes in the primary position and lids closed, place the probe tip on the lids, with the orientation marker upwards and the probe pointing slightly nasally.

4   For orientation, identify the concave curve of the posterior sclera and the optic nerve.

5   After thorough examination in the axial plane, reposition the probe to the limbus for transverse screening of the peripheral retina.

   ➤ If peripheral lesions are identified, proceed to longitudinal views, as described.

   ➤ Freeze any areas of interest on screen by pressing the foot pedal – these may then be printed out and/or the lesions measured using the caliper tool.

6   Kinetic examination will help distinguish structures and pathologies concerning the choroid/retina/vitreous interfaces.

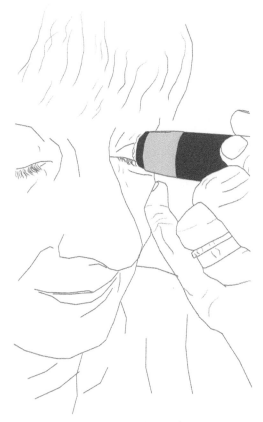

FIGURE PI5 Ensure the appropriate alignment of the probe

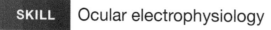

CODE: PI7

TARGET YEAR OF ACHIEVEMENT: 2

AIM: to understand electrodiagnostic tests (EDTs) pertaining to the assessment of the function of the retina and visual pathway, and to be able to interpret the results of such tests.

BACKGROUND

There are three components to electrodiagnostic testing: (1) electroretinography (ERG), (2) visual evoked potential (VEP) and (3) electrooculography (EOG). Each pertains to a separate part of the pathway. Before requesting EDTs, the clinician should have a clear idea of the possible diagnoses, particularly because the clear-cut diagnosis that one frequently hopes for from these investigations is seldom forthcoming – therefore, it is important to understand what you are hoping to ascertain from the test.

> Standards in electrophysiology are developed and updated by the International Society for Clinical Electrophysiology of Vision group. The techniques, reference ranges and best-practice guidelines produced by this group are available at www.iscev.org

ELECTRORETINOGRAPHY

ERG demonstrates electrical potential at the retina during stimulation. Corneal or lid electrodes are used to detect changes in electrical potential during and after stimulation of the neurosensory retina. Discrete populations of photoreceptors may be tested independently using scotopic (for rods) or photopic (for cones) stimuli. Flicker, pattern-reversal and coloured-flash stimuli are used to further isolate particular populations of photoreceptors. ERG is comprised of the A-wave, which corresponds to the photoreceptor layer, and the B-wave, which represents the electrical activity of the inner retinal layers.

ELECTROOCULOGRAPHY

EOG is used to establish retinal-pigment-epithelium (RPE) function. The eye functions electrically as a dipole, with the anode at the cornea and cathode at the retina. The potential difference between these two poles is measured by electrodes at the lateral and medial canthi. The subject is asked to look consecutively right and left – the differential electrical potential being picked up by the electrodes. To calculate RPE function, the eye must be dark adapted and the minimum resting potential recorded (the dark trough). This is compared with the maximum potential during photopic conditions (light peak). RPE function is calculated by dividing the light peak by the dark trough – giving the Arden ratio. The normal Arden ratio is greater than 1.8; diseases primarily affecting the RPE, such as Best's disease, demonstrate a reduced Arden ratio.

VISUAL EVOKED POTENTIAL

VEP testing interrogates the entire visual pathway, from the retina to the visual cortex, by using scalp-based electrodes. Thus, stimulation of the visual cortex is detected, and comparison of conduction times (since the time of stimulus is known) as well as the amplitudes of depolarisation form the VEP trace. VEPs are of particular use when the visual potential is unknown and the function of the optic pathways must be established.

The delay from light stimulation to the detection of activity is measured. The 'P100' is the delay from stimulation to the first positive cortical response after 100 ms. As it is assumed that the first 100 ms contain only background noise, they are excluded. The final value is averaged from many readings to reduce the effect of noise. P100 latencies of greater than 120 ms are generally considered pathological and are characteristically due to demyelination. The amplitude of the potential is of limited value, due to variations in recording techniques.

VEPs are generated in response to various stimuli. Comparison between these may be helpful because pattern (chequerboard) reversal tends to evoke a more powerful response than flash stimuli. However, response to the pattern-reversal target is degraded in the presence of uncorrected ametropia or media opacity, so comparison between the two will provide further information about the quality of image as well as conduction.

VEP records the function of the entire pathway – therefore, pathology cannot be localised without reference to EOG and ERG.

Biometry

CODE: PI12
TARGET YEAR OF ACHIEVEMENT: 2

BACKGROUND

While many intraocular-lens (IOL) manufacturers have extensive ranges of optics, including monofocal, multifocal, accommodating and toric implants, the first step in identifying the correct implant is to take accurate axial length (AL) and corneal-curvature measurements. Without these data, it is impossible to predict with any certainty the likely refractive outcome of surgery and, consequently, the benefit of that surgery.

Thus, biometry is a key pillar of modern cataract surgery. Although it is often carried out by nurses or other health professionals, it is imperative that trainees are versed not only in the interpretation of the results but also in the methods of acquisition.

There are two methods for the measurement of AL, although the most commonly employed device (the IOLMaster, Carl Zeiss Meditec, Germany) also incorporates corneal keratometry.

ULTRASOUND BIOMETRY

Previously the gold-standard technique for AL measurement, contact A-scan biometry is now reserved for those cases for which optical systems are not appropriate (dense cataract, corneal opacities). In contact A-scanning, the probe is placed on the anesthetised cornea and the distance from the probe and the echo from the RPE is measured. A contact A-scan trace demonstrates five spikes (cornea, anterior lens capsule, posterior lens capsule, RPE and sclera) in the phakic eye.

This is a simple test to undertake, and its results are generally adequate in most cases. The examiner must be careful not to compress the cornea with the probe, as this will result in an underestimation of AL, potentially resulting in an inappropriately high-powered lens choice. It should also be borne in mind that A-scan biometry tends to measure the anatomical AL, which may differ from the refractive AL (e.g. in posterior staphyloma).

Immersion A-scanning techniques provide much more reliable measurements and can be carried out relatively easily. A watertight shell is fitted over the probe, irrigating fluid runs through the shell and the entire device is placed over the anaesthetised eye. As the probe does not touch the cornea, there is no risk of compression. On average, immersion scanning ALs are 0.2 mm longer when compared with those obtained with contact techniques. Immersion A-scans display an extra anterior spike, representing the probe, in addition to the five standard spikes.

The corneal spike consists of two peaks (epithelium and endothelium); orientation with the visual axis is achieved when these two peaks are of the same amplitude. This is more easily observed with the immersion technique and provides more accurate biometry.

OPTICAL BIOMETRY

Modern biometric measurements are based on optical systems. These have a number of advantages over ultrasound systems: they are non-contact systems, so improve patient comfort, as well as accuracy; they often incorporate corneal keratometric measurement for the planning of astigmatic correction; and they can use multiple A-constants to provide a choice of lens to the surgeon.

Optical systems such as the IOLMaster use a partially coherent light wave to measure the distance from the tear film to the RPE. Typically, these systems take up to 10 measurements almost simultaneously then use the most statistically reliable result for the subsequent lens-power calculations.

While the acquisition of biometric data is straightforward, interpretation of the results is the key to ensuring good refractive outcomes.

A structured approach to interpreting biometric data

The output from an IOLMaster consists of three parts:
1 patient identifiers
2 refractive predictions
3 raw data from each measurement of each of the AL and corneal-curvature measurements as well as a graphical representation of the axial measurement.

It is important to establish whether the data pertain to the correct patient; their name, date of birth and unique hospital number will be printed in the top box. This should be checked and confirmed.

Check for consistency of AL measurements between each eye. When there is a significant difference, establish if this is due to anatomical/refractive reasons (e.g. posterior staphyloma, anisometropia) or measurement inconsistencies. Where the biometry data are unreliable they should be repeated.

RCOphth (2010) recommends that biometry should be repeated when:
- AL is <21.20 mm or >26.60 mm
- mean corneal power is <41 D or >47 D
- delta K is >2.5 D
- difference in AL between fellow eyes of >0.7 mm
- difference in mean corneal power of >0.9 nD.

The IOLMaster makes a number of individual AL measurements for each eye. The results of each of these should be checked next. Look for consistency of measurement. Beside each measurement, the signal-to-noise ratio (SNR) is displayed. Generally, the system will identify the value with the highest SNR as being the most reliable and base its IOL power calculations on this.

A number of keratometric (K) measurements are made, and, once again, the surgeon should ensure consistency in the readings. Inconsistent results suggest inaccuracy and should not be relied on. In this situation, either repeat the assessment, undertake separate corneal topography or disregard the corneal cylinder and aim for astigmatically neutral surgery. If efforts are made to correct the corneal cylinder during cataract surgery (on axis incisions, opposite clear corneal incisions or limbal-relaxing incisions) then the steep meridian must be identified and the chosen astigmatic corrective techniques employed with this in mind.

Summaries of the AL and K readings are provided as well as refractive predictions for up to four IOLs. These predictions are based on the A-constant of the given lens, the AL as measured and a mathematical formula.

Which formula?
- The RCOphth (2010) guidelines state that '[a]ll modern formulae perform well in the normal axial length range but the Haigis and Hoffer Q may be slightly better for short axial lengths'.
- Eyes in which photorefractive surgery (photorefractive keratectomy [PRK]/laser-assisted in situ keratomileusis [LASIK]/laser-assisted sub-epithelial keratectomy [LASEK]) has been performed require particular attention, and special calculations have been developed for use in these situations (e.g. Haigis-L).

A

Name: **H, JACK**
ID:
Date of birth: 16/03/1980
Age of patient: 34
Examination date: 30/04/2014
Surgeon: **Cardiff Eye Unit**
Lens: Alcon SA60AT

Target ref.: plano
n: 1.3375

AL measurements should be checked for plausibility as there may be pathological changes!

| **OD** right | AL: 23.61 mm (SNR = 386.4)
K1: 43.27 D / 7.80 mm @ 120°
K2: 43.55 D / 7.75 mm @ 30°
R / SE: 7.78 mm / 43.41 D
Cyl.: -0.28 D @ 120° | AL: 23.66 mm (SNR = 649.6)
K1: 43.27 D / 7.80 mm @ 28°
K2: 43.60 D / 7.74 mm @ 118°
R / SE: 7.77 mm / 43.44 D
Cyl.: -0.33 D @ 28° | **OS** left |

Refraction: 0 D 0 D @ 0°

Status: Phakic

Refraction: 0 D 0 D @ 0°

Status: Phakic

SRK®/T		Holladay 1		SRK®/T		Holladay 1	
A const:	118.80	SF:	1.67	A const:	118.80	SF:	1.67
IOL (D)	REF (D)	IOL (D)	REF (D)	IOL (D)	REF (D)	IOL (D)	REF (D)
22.5	-1.19	22.5	-1.19	22.0	-0.96	22.0	-0.98
22.0	-0.83	22.0	-0.84	21.5	-0.61	21.5	-0.63
21.5	-0.48	21.5	-0.49	21.0	-0.26	21.0	-0.28
21.0	**-0.13**	**21.0**	**-0.15**	**20.5**	**0.08**	**20.5**	**0.06**
20.5	0.21	20.5	0.19	20.0	0.42	20.0	0.40
20.0	0.55	20.0	0.53	19.5	0.76	19.5	0.73
19.5	0.88	19.5	0.86	19.0	1.09	19.0	1.06
Emme. IOL: 20.80		Emme. IOL: 20.78		Emme. IOL: 20.62		Emme. IOL: 20.59	

HofferQ		Haigis		HofferQ		Haigis	
pACD const:	5.44	A0 const: A1 const: A2 const:	-0.111 0.249 0.179	pACD const:	5.44	A0 const: A1 const: A2 const:	-0.111 0.249 0.179
IOL (D)	REF (D)	IOL (D)	REF (D)	IOL (D)	REF (D)	IOL (D)	REF (D)
22.5	-1.2			22.0	-1.0		
22.0	-0.8			21.5	-0.6		
21.5	-0.5			21.0	-0.3		
21.0	**-0.2**			**20.5**	**0.0**		
20.5	0.2			20.0	0.4		
20.0	0.5			19.5	0.7		
19.5	0.9			19.0	1.0		
Emme. IOL: 20.77				Emme. IOL: 20.56			

(* = value has been edited, ! = borderline value)

B

		Name: **H, JACK**	
		ID:	
		Date of birth: 16/03/1980	
		Examination date: 30/04/2014	n: 1.3375

AL measurements should be checked for plausibility as there may be pathological changes!

Axial length values

OD
right

OS
left

Phakic				Phakic			
Comp. AL: 23.61 mm		(SNR = 386.4)		Comp. AL: 23.66 mm		(SNR = 649.6)	
AL	SNR	AL	SNR	AL	SNR	AL	SNR
23.65 mm	5.8			23.67 mm	9.3		
23.43 mm	6.1			23.65 mm	4.2		
23.53 mm	6.2			23.64 mm	8.0		
23.54 mm	11.3			23.70 mm	8.5		
23.61 mm	11.1			23.66 mm	13.6		

Keratometer values

MV: 43.32/43.55 D	SD: 0.00 mm		MV: 43.27/43.60 D		SD: 0.01 mm	
---			K1: 43.21 D x 33°	7.81 mm	○ ○	
			K2: 43.60 D x 123°	7.74 mm	○ ○	
			ΔK: -0.39 D x 33°		✕ ○	
K1: 43.32 D x 117°	7.79 mm		K1: 43.21 D x 26°	7.81 mm	✕ ✕	
K2: 43.55 D x 27°	7.75 mm		K2: 43.55 D x 116°	7.75 mm	○ ○	
ΔK: -0.23 D x 117°			ΔK: -0.34 D x 26°		○ ✕	
K1: 43.27 D x 124°	7.80 mm		K1: 43.32 D x 27°	7.79 mm		
K2: 43.60 D x 34°	7.74 mm		K2: 43.60 D x 117°	7.74 mm		
ΔK: -0.33 D x 124°			ΔK: -0.28 D x 27°			

Anterior chamber depth values

White-to-white values

(* = value has been edited, ! = borderline value)

Carl Zeiss IOLMaster® Advanced Technology V. 7.7
Calibration checked on: 30/04/2014

Printed on: 30/04/2014 at 14:31.

FIGURE PI12A AND B IOLMaster biometer output

White-to-white (WTW) and anterior-chamber depth may be displayed on a biometry printout. These measurements are of use when anterior-chamber (angle-supported or iris-clip) implants are used.

When choosing a lens it makes sense to aim for low myopia in routine presbyopic patients. This should allow for good-quality general vision, particularly for everyday activities such as shopping, reading and conversation. Advise patients that they are likely to need glasses for reading and perhaps to improve their distance vision for activities such as driving.

Multifocal and accommodating IOLs are available, although, currently, their use is very limited in the public sector in which most trainees will be operating, and their use requires specific further training as well as scrupulous patient selection and management of post-operative expectations. Regardless of IOL selection, low myopes should be advised of the impact that aiming for emmetropia will have on any habitual unaided near vision.

It may be appropriate to intentionally aim for anisometropia in the form of monovision, leaving the patient with relative myopia in one eye and emmetropia in the fellow. This situation is not comfortable for all patients, so should be simulated with contact lenses prior to surgery.

REFERENCE

RCOphth. *Cataract Surgery Guidelines*. London: RCOphth; 2010. Available at: www.rcophth. ac.uk/core/core_picker/download.asp?id=544 (accessed 17 August 2014).

CODE: PI13
TARGET YEAR OF ACHIEVEMENT: 2

BACKGROUND

The 'visual field' is the extent and sensitivity of the area around fixation perceived by the visual system during fixation, and 'perimetry' is the study of this area. Visual fields are considered to represent the 'hill of vision', a mathematical representation of the varying sensitivities to luminance across the retina. The peak of the hill is found at the fovea, where sensitivity is highest, with reduced peripheral sensitivity demonstrated by the flatter 'foothills' towards the edges of the percept. The physiological scotoma created by the optic-nerve head is demonstrated by a gap in the hill, near its apex.

The ability of the visual system to perceive a target of a given luminance, size or velocity varies across the field. Therefore, it is important to establish the thresholds at which a given target will be perceived. This forms the basis of 'sub-threshold' testing, in which a target is provided that is initially not seen. As the variable being tested (luminance, size or velocity) is increased, the target becomes visible – this is the visual threshold for this particular target, at the retinal area being tested. Consecutive points across the retina of a given threshold can be mapped, producing a threshold contour – known as an 'isopter'.

'Suprathreshold' testing provides a target whose characteristics are consistently above the expected threshold for a given retinal location, and, as such, reduced or absent percept at this point is significant.

Visual stimuli for field testing may vary in their luminance, size or velocity. Perimetry using moving targets of uniform luminance and size is known as 'dynamic perimetry', and those tests using static targets of varying size or luminance are 'static' tests. In practice, the majority of testing undertaken in ophthalmic clinics is of the automated static type.

To fully interpret the results from a field test, it is important to bear in mind the neuronal arrangement within the retina, optic nerve, chiasm and optic tract.

- Retinal nerve fibres do not cross the horizontal midline.
- Fibres in the temporal retina arc above and below the horizontal midline raphe (arcuate fibres), while those from the nasal retina project radially to the optic-nerve head:
  - ➤ this gives rise to the characteristic field loss patterns of glaucoma – nasal-field loss patterns are the nasal step and arcuate scotoma, and temporal field loss patterns are the temporal wedge.
- Fibres nasal to the fovea (projecting temporal field) cross at the chiasm.
- The bundle of ipsilateral temporal retinal fibres and contralateral nasal fibres undergoes a 90-degree rotation within the optic tract.

CLINICAL APPLICATION

Objective measurements of peripheral-field perception can play an important role in the identification of pathology concerning the visual pathway as well as serving a role in the surveillance of disease over time.

Most patients are tested using automated machines, the use of which improves inter-test reliability. Various protocols exist; the clinician must select the correct one, and then be able to interpret the results.

Field-testing protocols for automated testing systems have been developed to improve the reliability of tests. Nomenclature concerns the origin of the protocol and the area and sensitivities tested. Common protocols for static perimetry include:

- Swedish interactive threshold algorithm (SITA): this is a family of tests, using a combination of threshold and suprathreshold stimuli. The test is adjusted to each patient's responses and provides a number of field types including:
  - ➤ SITA Standard
  - ➤ SITA Fast.
- FASTPAC:
  - ➤ these offer a reduced testing time compared with full-threshold testing
  - ➤ they are less accurate (there is no re-testing of missed points).

The area of field tested, and the number of points within that area, can be adjusted, with a balance being struck between accuracy and speed. Field testing depends on patient compliance and is rather tedious for them, requiring good motivation. Therefore, an accurate, fast test is preferred. The area being tested is important from the clinician's point of view: central fields are of interest for monitoring glaucomatous field loss, wider fields are used in suspected optic-pathway disease and binocular fields are relevant to driving vision.

Common testing patterns:
- 24–2: tests 54 points within the central 24 degree field (with points 6 degrees apart); this is the most common glaucoma screening field
- 30–2: tests 76 points within the central 30 degree field (points 6 degrees apart)
- 10–2: tests 68 points within a 10 degree field from fixation (points 2 degrees apart); this test is used in advanced glaucoma when the central field is threatened
- FF120: uniocular test of the field within 120 degrees of fixation; this is used for suspected neurological disease.

'Esterman driving fields' are binocular visual fields used in assessing the patient's ability to hold a driving licence (*see* Appendix for vision standards for driving, p. 129).

Indices and maps
- Reliability indices:
  - fixation losses – high rates of fixation loss suggest inattention
  - false-negative rate – should be less than 20%
  - false-positive rate – should be less than 10%.
- Analysis maps:
  - greyscale: the dominant map on the printout, this gives a global indication of threshold sensitivity across the field
  - numerical: this gives raw data on the sensitivity of each retinal point. Threshold values are given in decibels.
- Total deviation: a comparison of the field with a standard panel of age- and sex-matched fields.
- Pattern deviation: the total-deviation map after recalculation to take into account a generalised reduction in sensitivity. This is useful in the presence of media opacities.
- Probability indices: an indication of the significance of the field defect being present.
- Glaucoma hemifield test: a comparison of superior and inferior hemifield sensitivity – based on the assumption that there will be asymmetric reduction in sensitivity in early glaucoma.

Non-automated systems (Goldmann perimetry) are used more rarely than automated systems. Nevertheless, they have an important place in modern practice.

Goldmann perimetry provides threshold and suprathreshold kinetic perimetry. The user must set the luminance of the target and background as well as the size of the target.
- Target size is represented by Roman numerals 0–V.

- Target luminance is represented by Arabic numerals 1–4.
- Filter intensity is represented by lower-case letters (a = darkest, e = brightest).

Goldmann fields take longer to test and require a skilled perimetrist as well as a motivated patient. They are very useful in identifying subtle field defects either side of the vertical midline – a characteristic of neurological field loss and early scotoma – and for assessment in suspected cases of non-organic pathology in which there is apparent visual-field deficit that is not explained clinically. Classically, 'spiralling' fields are seen in non-organic pathology.

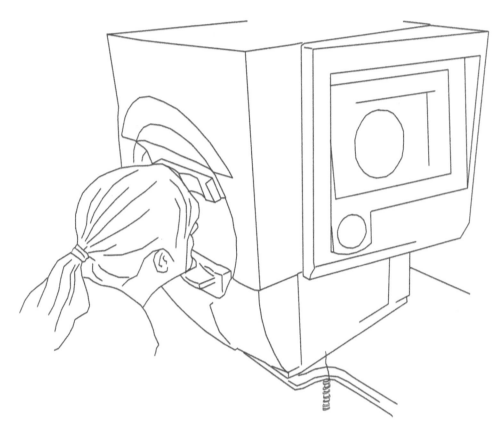

FIGURE PI13 Patient positioned at a Humphrey visual-field analyser

Practical skills

SKILL Periocular and intraocular drugs: intravitreal injection

CODE: PS3
TARGET YEAR OF ACHIEVEMENT: 7
AIM: to deliver intravitreal medication for the treatment of posterior-segment pathology.

BACKGROUND
Direct pharmacological treatment of posterior-segment pathology has undergone rapid development over the last 5 years. This approach now forms the mainstay of the treatment of exudative maculopathy related to choroidal neovascular membranes and will increasingly play a role in maculopathy related to diabetes and vascular disease. As the caseload continues to grow, it is the trainee Ophthalmologist who currently performs most of the intravitreal injections in most centres.

EQUIPMENT LIST
- Drug to be delivered in appropriate dose and concentration
- 27/30-gauge needle and 1 mL syringe
- Lid speculum, caliper and rule
- Local anaesthesia, dilating drops and surgical skin preparation
- Drape
- Topical antibiotic, pad and shield
- Cotton bud/Spear swab

CONSENT
- Purpose: to treat lesion, improve/stabilise vision.
- Serious or commonly occurring complications: loss of vision/blindness, endophthalmitis, cataract, pain, high pressure.

PROCEDURE
1 Check the patient's details, their consent and laterality of injection.
2 Dilate the pupil and anaesthetise the eye to be injected.
3 Undertake standard surgical preparation with forniceal povidone iodine, drape and speculum insertion.
4 Apply further topical anaesthetic drops and confirm anaesthesia with the tip of a needle.
5 An anaesthetic-soaked sterile cotton bud may be placed under the lid over the planned injection site. This should be left in place for at least 2 minutes.
6 Measure a distance of 3.5 mm (pseudophake) or 4.0 mm (phakic) from the surgical limbus using a preset gauge or caliper; light pressure with either device will leave an indent mark.
7 Place the needle tip on the indent mark and orientate the shaft towards the optic nerve.
8 Applying firm pressure will initially indent the globe, before some give is felt as the needle passes through the sclera and into the vitreous cavity. Advance the needle no more than 6 mm, and hold it in place with your non-dominant hand.
9 Slowly inject the drug then withdraw the needle, tamponading the site with a sterile cotton bud or spear swab.
10 Apply a topical antibiotic, pad and shield, as per local protocol.

Pearls

▶ Intravitreal preparations of more than 0.05 mL may cause a rise in intraocular pressure (IOP) sufficient to close the central retinal artery. This should be established by checking that the patient has hand-movements vision after the injection. Should there be a suggestion of reduced vision, the central artery can be checked with an indirect ophthalmoscope and 20D lens. If the artery is not perfused, an anterior-chamber paracentesis should be performed (*see* PS9, p. 74).

▶ The most common site for injection is the superotemporal quadrant. Other sites may be used to avoid scleromalacia with repeated injections.

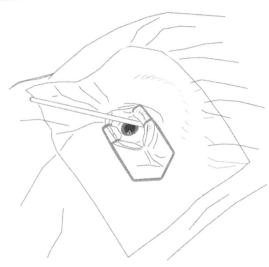

FIGURE PS3.1A Place a cotton bud soaked in topical anaesthetic under the lid in the position of the planned injection

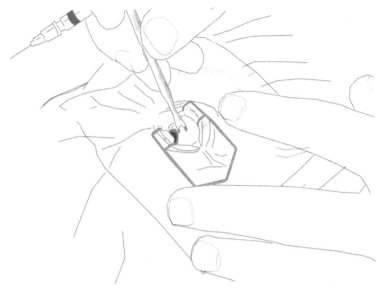

FIGURE PS3.1B Mark the injection site as measured from the limbus (3.5 mm for pseudophakes; 4.0 mm for phakic patients)

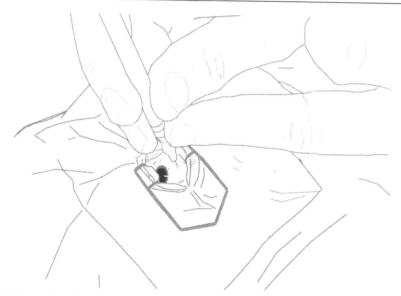

FIGURE PS3.1C The injection should be delivered to a depth of around 6 mm, with the needle orientated towards the posterior pole

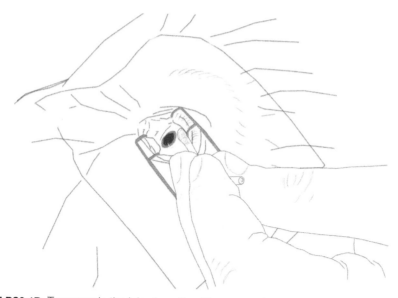

FIGURE PS3.1D Tamponade the injection site with a cotton bud

Periocular and intraocular drugs: orbital-floor/peribulbar injection

CODE: PS3

TARGET YEAR OF ACHIEVEMENT: 7

AIM: to deliver drugs to the extraconal space inferior to the globe. Both steroid and anaesthetic agents may be delivered via this route.

EQUIPMENT LIST
- Drug to be delivered
- Syringe (2 mL) and 25 gauge needle
- Povidone iodine/Chlorhexidine skin preparation
- Topical anaesthetic drops
- Chloramphenicol ointment
- Double pad

CONSENT
- Purpose 1 – orbital-floor steroid: to reduce retinal oedema, control inflammation, and improve vision.
- Serious or commonly occurring complications: globe injury/perforation, reduced vision, retrobulbar haemorrhage, orbital fat atrophy.

- Purpose 2 – peribulbar anaesthesia: to provide anaesthesia and akinesia for surgery.
- Serious and commonly occurring side effects: globe injury/perforation, loss of vision/blindness, orbital haemorrhage/haematoma.

PROCEDURE
The approach may be either conjunctival – via the inferior fornix – or through the skin of the lower lid.
1 Instil topical anaesthesia.
2 Disinfect the conjunctival sac and skin using povidone iodine.
3 Ask the patient to look up, and identify the inferior orbital notch.
4 Pass the needle, bevel up, over the inferior orbital notch, and aim inferiorly and medially – towards the contralateral occipital condyle.
5 The needle tip should follow the periosteum of the orbital floor.
6 Confirm the location of the needle is inferior to the globe by asking the patient to look down and then up – the needle should not move.
7 Pass around two-thirds of the length of the needle; there is no need to pass it to the hilt.
8 Aspirate to confirm the tip has not pierced a vessel.
9 Deliver the drug slowly and smoothly.
10 Remove the needle and apply pressure through gauze.

INTRA-OPERATIVE CONSIDERATION
- If globe rupture is suspected, remove the needle and syringe, and seek senior advice immediately.

POST-OPERATIVE CONSIDERATIONS
- This is generally a painless procedure, but the patient may complain of a mild ache afterwards.
- Orbital haemorrhage/haematoma is a rare complication that may cause non-axial proptosis or diplopia.

SKILL Local anaesthesia

CODE: PS5
TARGET YEAR OF ACHIEVEMENT: 3
AIM: to establish local anaesthesia for ocular surgery.

BACKGROUND

Adequate local anaesthesia makes modern-day ophthalmic surgery possible. Local anaesthesia in ophthalmic practice is in routine use for both extra- and intraocular surgery.

Lid surgery may require intra- and sub-dermal as well as periosteal infiltration.

Most intraocular surgery is performed with the patient under either topical anaesthesia, sub-Tenon's blockade or peribulbar blockade. The historical use of retrobulbar injections has been almost entirely superseded by the safer peribulbar approach. Subconjunctival and topical anaesthesia for cataract surgery provide excellent analgesia but give no akinesia – thus, a compliant patient is important; analgesia may be augmented during surgery with further topical or intra-cameral anaesthetic.

GENERAL NOTES ON LOCAL ANAESTHESIA

The use of adrenaline in local anaesthetics used for sub-Tenon's or peribulbar anaesthesia is contraindicated to avoid vasospasm of the central retinal artery (the retina has no collateral circulation). Conversely, adrenaline is very useful for skin anaesthesia, as it reduces bleeding; however, greater volumes of anaesthetic are required when adrenaline is used.

Local anaesthetics are painful. This can be reduced by:
- warming the anaesthetic
- buffering the pH
- injecting slowly.

It is less painful to make a single needle tract, infiltrating as you go, than a number of separate injection points. If you infiltrate anaesthetic as the needle is advanced, the tip will be preceded by a wave of anaesthetic, reducing discomfort to the patient.

Mark the skin prior to infiltrating. It is difficult to plan surgical incisions after infiltration, as the skin's contours, volumes and relations are distorted. When possible, use permanent ink to mark incisions. If a water-soluble ink such as gentian violet is used, dry well before infiltrating the anaesthetic.

Anaesthetic fluid infiltrated along tissue planes may be used to develop the planes of the lid, making subsequent dissection simpler.

Local anaesthetic agents may induce dysrhythmia. Patients undergoing topical anaesthesia should be monitored and appropriate resuscitation resources must be available.

EXTRAOCULAR ANAESTHESIA
Dermal, sub-dermal and periosteal anaesthesia
Clinical context

These are used for most lid surgery, as well as the correction of entropion with everting sutures. The choice of anaesthetic agent will depend on the procedure to be undertaken.

Some commonly used periocular anaesthetics:
- 2% lignocaine with 1:80 000 adrenaline (Lignospan Special™)
- levobupivacaine (5 mg/mL) (Chirocaine™).

Procedure

The key to comfortable anaesthesia is patient compliance. Take care to keep the needle and syringe out of the patient's sight if possible. Ensure topical anaesthesia has been instilled, and plan the injection before carrying it out.

1 Apply traction to the lid, away from the planned entry of the needle.
2 Ask the patient to look away from the injection site to reduce the risk of globe injury.
3 Control the direction of the needle with the angle of entry and the position of the syringe, always imagining the position of the needle within the tissue. Never push a needle through tissue towards your own finger.
4 Aspirate before injecting, and slowly inject as the needle tip is advanced.

Periosteal anaesthesia

Surgery of the lateral canthus and lateral orbital rim is commonly undertaken to correct both entropion and ectropion. As well as lid anaesthesia, good anaesthesia of the insertion of the lateral canthal tendon is required.

Procedure

1 Identify the lateral orbital rim by palpation, distracting the lateral canthal angle laterally.
2 Place the needle directly through the conjunctiva, vertically towards the palpated position of the rim.
3 The needle tip will be felt to engage the periosteum. Inject at this site, continuing to infiltrate as the needle is withdrawn.

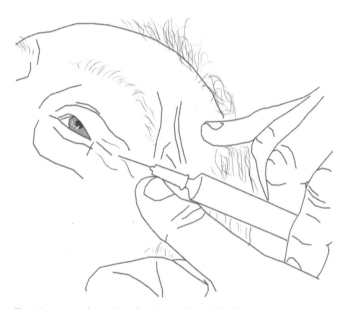

FIGURE PS5.1 Traction away from the direction of the injection

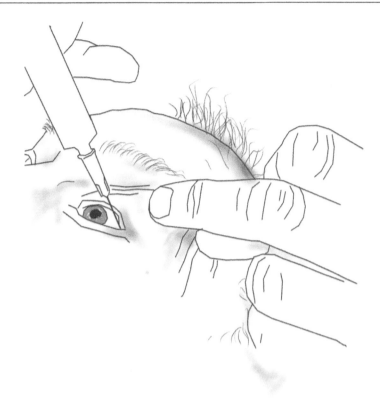

FIGURE PS5.2 Periosteal infiltration

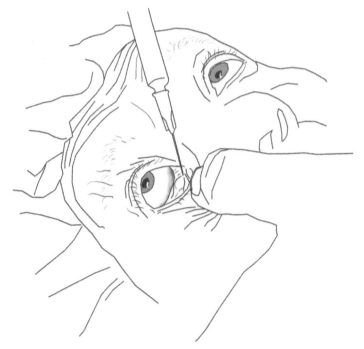

FIGURE PS5.3 Sub-conjunctival injection. The patient should look away from the needle. (Injection may be within the tarsal conjunctiva, as demonstrated here, or within the bulbar conjunctiva)

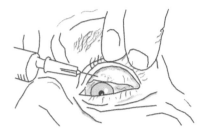

FIGURE PS5.4 Sub-tarsal injection. Ensure secure lid eversion, and rest the syringe on the bridge of the nose

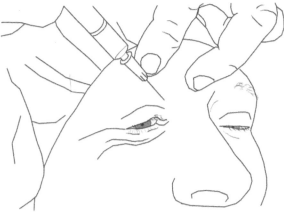

FIGURE PS5.5 Stabilise the area to be injected, and avoid inadvertent inoculation injury during injection

SUB-TENONS ANAESTHESIA
Equipment list
- Topical anaesthesia
- Lid speculum
- Lignocaine (2%) ± 0.75 mg/mL Chirocaine
- Sub-Tenon's cannula
- Moorfields forceps and Westcott scissors

Anatomical consideration
- 'Tenon's capsule' is a fibrous coat between the bulbar conjunctiva and the sclera. It inserts around 1.5 mm posterior to the surgical limbus and is loosely attached to the sclera.

Procedure
1 Instil topical anaesthesia and place the speculum.
2 Tent the infero-nasal conjunctiva 2–3 mm from the limbus with the forceps, and make a single cut into the sub-Tenon's space.
3 Bluntly dissect this space using the Westcott scissors, aiming posteriorly between the medial and inferior recti and deep to the inferior oblique.
4 Insert the Tenon's cannula into this space, approximately 4 cm posteriorly, following the curve of the globe.
5 Retract the cannula until it is firmly opposed to the posterior globe then infiltrate the local anaesthesia.
6 Confirm motor blockade prior to surgery.

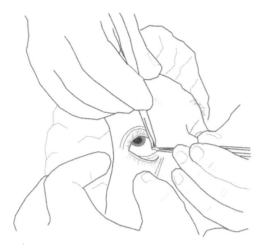

FIGURE PS5.6 Tent the infero-nasal conjunctiva 2–3 mm from the limbus, then open and develop the sub-conjunctival space with Westcott scissors

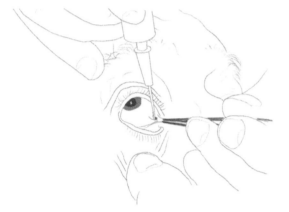

FIGURE PS5.7 Introduce the cannula, with the curve against the globe

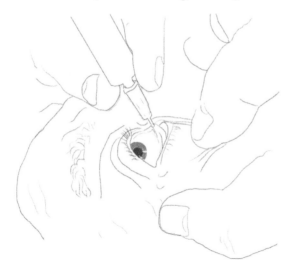

FIGURE PS5.8 Introduce the cannula posteriorly, before retracting it until firm apposition against the poster curve of the globe is felt. Slowly infiltrate in this position

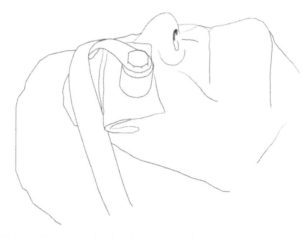

FIGURE PS5.9 Protect the eye by taping it closed and applying a pad and weight to distribute the anaesthetic

CODE: PS6
TARGET YEAR OF ACHIEVEMENT: 7
AIM: to use an electrical current to establish haemostasis and/or permanent scarring.

BACKGROUND

Units may be 'monopolar' or 'bipolar'. The current in monopolar cautery travels through the tissue, in bipolar cautery it travels across the tissue. Monopolar units require a skin plate as the second electrode (the first being at the tip of the instrument) and tend to be more destructive and less precise. Bipolar units comprise forceps, where the tips are the electrodes. The tissue can be grasped then cauterised easily, and the effect confined to the area between the tips.

Most units use bipolar diathermy for haemostasis. Monopolar 'cutting cautery' may be used in oculoplastic practice, frequently as a disposable 'hot-rod' high-resistance wire loop.

SAFETY CONSIDERATIONS

- Bipolar cautery is generally safe, as the effect is local and dependent on the electrical resistance of the tissue being cauterised.
- Monopolar and 'hot-rod' cautery should never be used in the presence of piped oxygen, due to the risk of arcing and ignition. Care should be taken to remove all dry swabs from the surgical field when using high-resistance cutting cautery.
- Monopolar skin plates should be placed on the contralateral side from any metallic prostheses such as hip or knee implants.
- Monopolar cautery will cut through most tissues quickly and cleanly. Extreme care should therefore be exercised when using such instruments close to the globe or when dissecting through tissue planes.

Cryotherapy

CODE: PS7

This skill no longer appears in the RCOphth curriculum but remains an important skill with which to be familiar.

AIM: to permanently remove lashes from the lid to prevent ongoing trichiatic damage to the ocular surface.

EQUIPMENT LIST

- Lignocaine (2%) and 1:80 000 adrenaline, with syringe and grey needle
- Cryotherapy probe – lid probe
- Sterile irrigation fluid (balanced salt solution)

CONSENT

- Purpose: to permanently remove lashes.
- Serious or commonly occurring complications: permanent loss of lashes, scarring causing lid malposition and subsequent surgery, recurrence of lashes.

PROCEDURE

- Infiltrate local anaesthesia into the lid margin and adjacent lid.
- Confirm the function of the cryo probe – a frost ball should form on the plate.
- Place the heel of the cryo probe onto the lash line.
- Ensure no contact is made with the conjunctiva.
- Complete two freeze–thaw cycles to a temperature of –20 degrees Celsius.
  - ➤ For upper-lid lashes, use 25-second cycles.
  - ➤ For lower-lid lashes, use 20-second cycles.
- Remove the devitalised lashes after at least a week following the procedure.

Pearl

▌ Damage to the lash roots occurs during thawing, so this process this should not be sped up. There is frequently an acceleration of lash growth after cryotherapy – this lasts 5 days. When this occurs, it may be necessary to perform manual epilation.

CODE: PS8
TARGET YEAR OF ACHIEVEMENT: 2

CLINICAL CONTEXT

Dry-eye disease represents a significant proportion of the caseload in eye departments. Dry-eye disease may be due to:

- tear factors:
  - ➤ incompetent mucinous phase – goblet-cell dysfunction (Stevens–Johnson syndrome, post traumatic)
  - ➤ hyposecretion of the aqueous phase – autoimmune connective-tissue disease (Sjögren's syndrome, rheumatoid arthritis)
  - ➤ unstable lipid phase – hyper-/hyposecretion (meibomian gland dysfunction [MGD]).
- lid factors:
  - ➤ lid malposition – ectropion/entropion
  - ➤ lid-margin irregularity (post-surgical steps and notches)
  - ➤ cicatricial lid disease (ocular cicatricial pemphigoid, chronic staphylococcal lid disease).
- drainage factors (while the following are causes of epiphora rather than dry eye, an adequate assessment of tear-film dynamics should include the assessment of tear drainage):
  - ➤ nasolacrimal duct obstruction
  - ➤ canalicular obstruction
  - ➤ punctal stenosis.

The clinician must identify:
- the severity of the disease
- the cause of the dysfunction
- any systemic associations.

Assessment of severity is based on symptoms and signs. A thorough examination of the ocular surface should be undertaken, with particular attention paid to any evidence of corneal epithelial disease.

TESTING OF EACH CAUSATIVE FACTOR
A basic examination

Due to the subtle nature of the tear film, it is vital to assess it using the least invasive methods first. In particular, bright slit-lamp light will cause reflex aqueous secretion, so must be avoided initially. When irritated eyes are mentioned during history taking, it is important to watch how the patient habitually blinks while in conversation, as rapid blinking can be a good indication of ocular discomfort. History taking should incorporate an assessment of aqueous deficiency, including Sjögren's syndrome, and a question to determine ocular involvement may be asked – that is, the ease of reflex tearing when chopping onions/emotionally upset. In addition, questioning about other mucosal areas is important (e.g. does the patient habitually require a drink to aid swallowing toast or biscuits? Has the female patient suffered from excessive vaginal dryness? Has the patient suffered from recurrent epistaxis?).

It is sensible to first examine the corneal tear film on slit-lamp examination without fluorescein, using a thin, mid-bright white beam that has been adjusted on skin to the correct size and illumination. Note if excessive lipid is present (suggestive of MGD) or debris (suggestive of poor quality make-up or its removal).

An examination of the lower and upper lid margins for apposition, laxity, hyperaemia and meibomian gland abnormalities is important. Any notches should be explored by lid eversion. Notching indicating meibomian gland drop-out is associated with a poor level of lipid expression, decreased ocular lubrication and increased ocular evaporation. Eighty per cent of dry eye is evaporative and may be treated with ocular beanbag heat packs, to encourage natural gland expression, and/or lipid-replacement sprays.

Sodium fluorescein (not in conjunction with an anaesthetic) is useful to assess corneal and conjunctival epithelia involvement and the severity of the ocular-surface defect. Its use for tear-film break-up time (TBUT) is limited due to the artificial increase in aqueous levels created and the disruption of the overlying lipid layer as the sodium fluorescein binds to the aqueous layer. Excessive staining indicates that the overlying mucin layer is damaged. Lissamine™ Green is useful to assess for lid-wiper epitheliopathy on the tarsal conjunctiva, particularly in contact-lens wearers, in whom lens surface friction has caused damage around the inner lid margin – this can be avoided by using a biocompatible lens and ocular lubricants.

Expression of the meibomian glands is useful diagnostically. The examiner's thumb, held over the lid margin, slowly and gently compresses the meibomian glands under the lower eyelid; expression of transparent oil in at least two-thirds of glands should be noted. Variations in oil secretion are likely to be found in MGD.

A comprehensive examination: overview
- Tear factors:
  - ➤ mucin: rose bengal staining to identify areas of poor mucin production
  - ➤ aqueous phase: Schirmer's test and fluorescein meniscus time (FMT)
  - ➤ lipid phase: TBUT.
- Lid factors:
  - ➤ examine the position of the lid margin and lashes to identify malposition
  - ➤ assess horizontal lid laxity, the competence of lower-lid retractors and the position of fornices.
- Drainage factors:
  - ➤ fluorescein dye disappearance test (FDDT) and modified Jones test
  - ➤ lacrimal-sac reflux testing
  - ➤ sac washout/probing.

A comprehensive examination: detailed notes
Rose bengal
'Rose bengal' is a rarely used topical dye which stains areas of conjunctiva with poorly functioning or absent goblet cells. Its adherence to healthy cells is blocked by mucin. Rose bengal stings on instillation and is seldom found in clinic.

Schirmer's testing of basal tear production (Schirmer's test 1)
Procedure
1 Place a strip of filter paper (number 41 Whatman paper) into the anaesthetised inferior fornix.
2 Ask the patient to gently close their eyes and keep them closed for around 5 minutes.
3 Measure the extent of tear wetting:
  - ➤ less than 5 mm suggests aqueous hyposecretion
  - ➤ 5–10 mm is borderline.

Schirmer's testing of reflex tear production (Schirmer's test 2)
Procedure
The procedure for Schirmer's test 2 is the same as for Schirmer's test 1, but the nasal mucosa should be stimulated during testing.

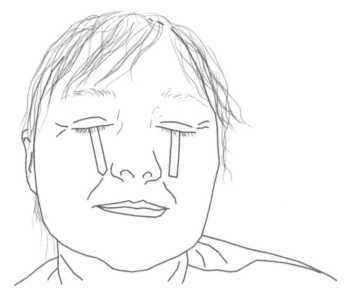

FIGURE PS8.1 Schirmer's test

Fluorescein tear tests
These are four useful tests which may be carried out consecutively using a single drop of 2% fluorescein:
- FMT
- TBUT
- FDDT
- Jones test.

Procedure
1 Instruct the patient to look up and not to squeeze their eyes.
2 Pull the lower lid down, with your finger pressing on the superior maxilla.
3 Instil a single drop of 2% fluorescein in the centre of the inferior fornix.
4 **FMT:** assess time taken for fluorescence to occur at the pupillary midline:
   ➤ more than 3 minutes suggests aqueous hyposecretion
   ➤ less than 1 minute suggests hypersecretion, which may be reflex.
5 **TBUT:** ask the patient to blink, then examine the corneal surface with broad, bright cobalt blue illumination while holding the upper lid.
   ➤ Dark streaks or spots will appear as the lipid phase breaks down, allowing evaporation of the tear.
   ➤ A normal TBUT is around 10 seconds. Very rapid break-up (less than 5 seconds) suggests incompetent lipid phase.
6 **FDDT:** assess the height of the tear film under cobalt blue light then re-examine the tear-film position 13 minutes after instillation of the dye.
   ➤ Persistence of dye in the meniscus implies nasolacrimal duct obstruction.
   — Ensure that the patient does not dab their eye dry during testing.
7 The test can be used in infants, in which presence of fluorescence in the oropharynx confirms patent drainage (modified **Jones test**).

Syringing of the lacrimal canaliculi
Procedure
1 Instil topical anaesthesia.
2 Dilate the punctae with a Nettleship dilator if stenosis is present.
  ➤ Engage the punctum with the tip of the dilator before passing it inferomedially and maintaining firm lateral traction on the lid.
3 Pass a nasolacrimal cannula, mounted on a 2 mL syringe containing NaCl solution, vertically through the punctum.
4 Follow the course of the canaliculus, inferiorly 2 mm, then medially.
  ➤ There should be minimal resistance to progress along the canaliculus.
5 When the tip is in the distal canaliculus, gently inject fluid.
  ➤ Reflux through the cannulated punctum indicates a blockage within that canaliculus.
6 Reflux through the un-cannulated punctum indicates common canalicular or lacrimal-sac blockage.
  ➤ A patent system is demonstrated by the patient's sensation of fluid in the throat.
  ➤ If blockage distal to the common canaliculus is suspected, the ducts may be probed (*see following*).

Probing of lacrimal drainage ducts
1 This is an uncomfortable procedure for patients, and general anaesthesia is essential.
2 Dilate the punctum with Nettleship dilator.
3 Pass as wide a probe as possible into the sac using the same technique as for syringing.
  ➤ Assess for:
    — hard stop: the tip of the probe is pushed against the periosteum of the lacrimal bone, indicating its presence in the sac. If a hard stop is felt:
      i reorientate the heel of the probe medially, so that the tip is directed towards the duct
      ii pass it inferiorly, into the nose, to confirm a patent system.
    — soft stop: the tip of the probe does not make contact with the periosteum, indicating a blockage within the canaliculus/common canaliculus.

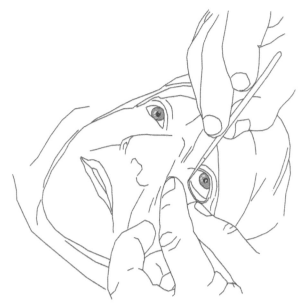

FIGURE PS8.2 Dilate the punctum with a Nettleship dilator. Apply tight lateral traction to the lid to stabilise the punctum

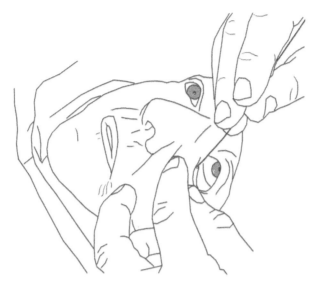

FIGURE PS8.3 Pass the probe inferiorly 2 mm, while applying lateral lid traction

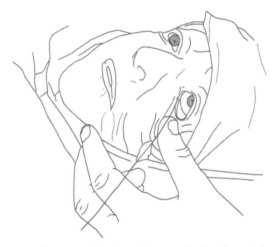

FIGURE PS8.4 Pass the probe smoothly down the canaliculus. Do not force the probe tip past obstructions, and assess the quality of the stop within the sac

Anterior-chamber paracentesis

CODE: PS9
TARGET YEAR OF ACHIEVEMENT: 7
AIM: to reduce IOP to allow refilling of the central retinal artery in the context of CRAO of less then 2 hours' duration.

CONSENT
- Purpose: to attempt to improve vision by reperfusing the central retinal artery.
- Serious or commonly occurring complications: damage to ocular structures including iris stroma and anterior lens capsule, hypotony, choroidal effusion, endophthalmitis, loss of vision.

EQUIPMENT LIST
- Slit-lamp biomicroscope
- Insulin syringe and needle
- Topical anaesthesia
- Povidone iodine
- Topical antibiotics
- Double pad

ANATOMICAL CONSIDERATIONS
- Paracentesis is made just anterior to the limbus.
- Iris injury is more likely in hyperopic eyes and iris bombe.
- Inoculation of eyelid flora is less likely if paracentesis is made temporally.

PHYSIOLOGICAL CONSIDERATIONS
- The procedure is indicated in CRAO of less than 2 hours.
- There is increased risk of suprachoroidal effusion in hypertensives.

PROCEDURE
1 Ensure patient comfort at the slit lamp.
2 Instil topical anaesthesia with/without povidone iodine.
3 Remove the plunger from the syringe.
4 Introduce the needle temporally, with its bevel anteriorly to avoid iris incarceration.
5 Ensure a long intrastromal tract.
6 Make sure the needle stays within the anterior chamber, and observe the droplets of aqueous passing into the barrel of the syringe.
7 Remove the needle along the same track.
8 Further aqueous may be 'burped' from the wound by exerting light pressure on the limbal sclera.
9 Instil antibiotic drops and pad the eye.

Corneal scrape

CODE: PS10
TARGET YEAR: 2
AIM: to debride corneal epithelium/anterior stromal tissue to provide diagnosis and improve local drug delivery.

EQUIPMENT LIST
- Topical anaesthesia
- Size 11 blade
- Suture-tying forceps
- Green/Orange needle mounted on a 5 mL syringe
- Microbiology transport medium/plates
- Topical antibiotics

PROCEDURE
1. Ensure adequate topical anaesthesia.
2. Explain to the patient that it is important that they keep their forehead pushed against the headband.
3. Rest the heel of your dominant hand on the patient's brow, supporting the elbow on the slit-lamp desk and approach the eye from the side.
4. Face the bevel of the needle away from the globe, or, if using the blade, make sure it is perpendicular to the corneal surface.
5. Choose an area of healthy epithelium adjacent to the area to be scraped and lift it with the needle or blade tip.
6. Using either the needle or blade tip, or the forceps, debride a generous area of epithelium around the lesion.
7. Wash off into the transport medium or a plate, directly onto agar.
8. Explore deeper lesions with care using the blade tip, taking care not to re-inoculate the lesion with the instrument – change the needle/blade between visits to the eye.
9. Instil topical antibiotics and warn the patient of discomfort due to epithelial defect.
10. Record the extent of the epithelial defect after scraping.

Ocular-surface foreign body

CODE: PS11
TARGET YEAR OF ACHIEVEMENT: 1
AIM: to safely remove embedded foreign material from the ocular surface.

EQUIPMENT LIST

- Topical anaesthesia
- Orange needle mounted on 5 mL syringe *or* Algerbrush with burr
- Fluorescein sodium (1%–2%)
- Tropicamide (1%)
- Phenylephrine (2.5%)
- Bandage contact lens (*see* PS14, p. 80)

PROCEDURE

1 Establish the depth of the embedded particle using a narrow, bright beam and oblique illumination.
2 Instil adequate volume of topical anaesthesia.
3 Support the heel of your dominant hand on the patient's brow or the headband of the slit lamp and your elbow with the slit-lamp table/bolster.
4 Approach the eye from the side, and confirm to the patient the importance of pressing firmly on the headband.
5 Using the needle tip undermine the edge of the foreign body, and work to a point behind it, then flick outwards to dislodge the particle.
6 Rust rings may be removed using a circular scraping movement with the needle, or alternatively with the Algerbrush and burr.
7 Establish the integrity of the wound using 1%–2% fluorescein sodium and Seidel test.

NOTES

- Any high-velocity projectile may cause a penetrating injury. Therefore, all such cases, including those involving metal fragments from grinding and welding incidents, should be adequately dilated and an extensive posterior-segment examination carried out.
- Features of penetrating injury include:
  ➤ leaking corneal wound
  ➤ low IOP or shallowed anterior chamber
  ➤ sub-conjunctival haemorrhage extending into the fornix
  ➤ iris bleed or transillumination defect
  ➤ vitreous haemorrhage.
- A leak should be tamponaded with a bandage contact lens and senior advice sought.
  ➤ Most small leaks will close spontaneously, and the aim of management is to prevent infection and hypotony.

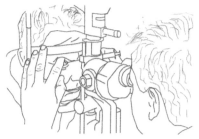

FIGURE PS11.1 Both the patient and clinician should be comfortable at the slit lamp

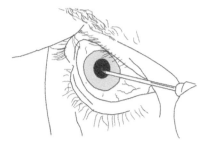

FIGURE PS11.2 Firmly hold upper lid on to the superior orbital rim, and undermine the foreign body using the needle tip

Occlude nasolacrimal puncta

CODE: PS12
TARGET YEAR OF ACHIEVEMENT: 7
AIM: to temporarily occlude the nasolacrimal puncta to improve the retention of the tear film.

EQUIPMENT LIST
- Topical anaesthesia
- Punctal plug of appropriate size
- Nettleship punctal dilator

PROCEDURE
1 Ensure adequate topical anaesthesia.
2 Apply lateral traction to the lid to stabilise the punctum.
3 Dilate the punctum with the integrated or Nettleship dilator.
4 Push the plug into the punctum, until the tip of the applicator is level with the lid margin.
5 Squeeze the applicator to deploy the plug.

Pearls
- Punctal plugs are available in various sizes. Use the largest plug that can be injected to ensure it will be retained.
- If a patient does not get troublesome epiphora with plugs, it may be worthwhile considering permanent punctal occlusion with cautery.
- Punctal plugs increase the risk of ocular-surface infection, so, ideally, should not be used for both the upper and lower punctae on one side. The patient should be warned to seek help if they develop symptoms suggestive of conjunctivitis or keratitis.

Remove corneal sutures

CODE: PS13

TARGET YEAR OF ACHIEVEMENT: 2

AIM: to safely remove corneal sutures following corneal graft or corneal repair

EQUIPMENT LIST
- Topical anaesthesia
- Suture-tying forceps
- Orange needle mounted on a 3 or 5 mL syringe *or* Vannas scissors

PROCEDURE
1 Ensure adequate topical anaesthesia.
2 Identify the sutures to be removed.
3 Undermine the superficial pass of the suture using the needle tip or scissor blade on the host side of the interface.
4 Cut the suture using the sharp edge of the needle bevel or scissors.
5 Mobilise the long end of the suture, and re-grasp just above the point where it enters the cornea.
6 Remove the suture using a swift movement towards the centre of the cornea, in line with the direction of the suture.

NOTES
- When planning suture removal for astigmatic correction, up-to-date corneal topography and refraction are helpful.
- To relieve corneal astigmatism, sutures on the steep meridian should be removed. (The astigmatism will be increased if sutures on the flat meridian are removed.)
- If the patient has no significant corneal astigmatism following penetrating keratoplasty or deep anterior lamellar keratoplasty, alternate sutures may be removed.
- If a single continuous suture is to be removed, it may be cut at each superficial throw and treated as interrupted sutures.

Fit a bandage contact lens

CODE: PS14
TARGET YEAR OF ACHIEVEMENT: 3
AIM: to safely and comfortably place a contact lens for protection of the ocular surface.

EQUIPMENT LIST
- Bandage contact lens
- Gallipot
- Sterile saline
- Non-toothed forceps (Moorfields)

PROCEDURE
A bandage contact lens may be inserted using a fingertip or forcep.

Instillation by fingertip
1 Ensure your hands are clean.
2 Check the expiry date and serial number of the contact lens.
3 Pour the contents of the lens bottle into the gallipot and identify the lens.
4 Explain the procedure to the patient then recline them to 45 degrees.
5 Instil topical anaesthesia and ask patient to look up.
6 Pick the lens up on its anterior (convex) surface with the tip of a finger of your dominant hand.
7 Ensure the patient's lids are retracted and the entire cornea is exposed.
8 Place the lens onto the ocular surface with a rolling motion to reduce the size of the bubble behind the lens.
9 Ask the patient to blink to check security of the lens.

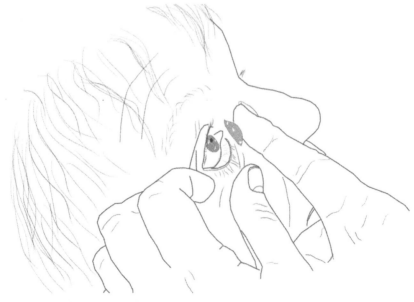

FIGURE PS14 Bandage contact lens insertion

Forceps technique

1 Undertake Steps 1–5 of the 'Instillation by hand' procedure.
2 Use a pair of non-toothed forceps, such as Moorfields, to pick up the edge of the lens.
3 Place the lens onto the anaesthetised ocular surface, then unfold it using the closed tip of the forceps.
4 Ask the patient to blink to check security of the lens.

Administer periocular botulinum toxin

CODE: PS15
TARGET YEAR OF ACHIEVEMENT: 7

BACKGROUND
'Botulinum toxin' is an inhibitor of cholinergic neuromuscular transmission. It results in blockade of the neuromuscular junction which may last for up to 3 months.

Which preparation?
Two preparations are available:
● Botox®
● Dysport®.

In general the dose ratio between Dysport and Botox is 4:1.

Dose for hemifacial spasm and blepharospasm
Twenty units of Dysport in three sites within pre-tarsal skin or orbicularis.

Dose for induction of upper lid ptosis
Twenty to 40 units Dysport or five to 10 units Botox.

Dose for crocodile tears
Five units of Botox into the lacrimal gland.

Dose for treatment of paralytic ectropion
Twenty units of Dysport into orbicularis.

CLINICAL APPLICATION
Botulinum toxin is used for the treatment of facial dystonias and hemifacial spasm. It may also be used to produce a ptosis for protection of the ocular surface (*see* SS8, p. 93), or, when injected into extraocular muscles, may control some forms of strabismus causing diplopia.

TREATMENT OF HEMIFACIAL SPASM AND BLEPHAROSPASM
Consent
● Purpose: control of muscle twitching.
● Serious or commonly occurring complications: progressive loss of muscle tone with repeated injections, reduced facial expression, bruising/bleeding, infection.

Procedure
1 Identify the dystonic muscle.
  ➤ The orbicularis is most common, but the frontalis may also be involved.
2 Identify the nodal points for the twitch, and aim to inject these sites.
3 Make each injection sub-dermally, raising a small bleb at each point.

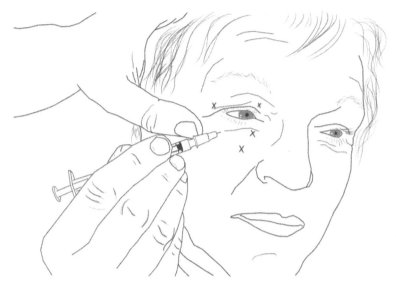

FIGURE PS15 The position of the injection should be tailored to the affected muscles

INDUCTION OF UPPER-LID PTOSIS
Consent
- Purpose: protection of the ocular surface.
- Serious or commonly occurring complications: worsening of exposure (through SR paresis), failure of ptosis, cosmetically apparent facial asymmetry/ptosis.

Procedure
1 Ask the patient to look down to the floor.
2 Identify the upper-lid skin crease.
3 Pass the needle through the lid, just superior to the lid crease below the brow, and superior orbital margin, nasal to the superior orbital notch, aiming upwards towards the roof of the orbit.
4 Using a short orange needle, pass the needle to the hilt.
5 Ask the patient to look up and down to confirm the needle tip's position outside of the muscle cone.
6 Aspirate before injecting as the needle is withdrawn.

Pearls
▶ Avoid injecting the SR, as doing so will obliterate Bell's phenomenon and may exacerbate corneal exposure.
▶ It may take a day or two for the ptosis to complete – in the meantime, the surface must be protected with simple measures such as tape or a temporary tarsorrhaphy (p. 94).

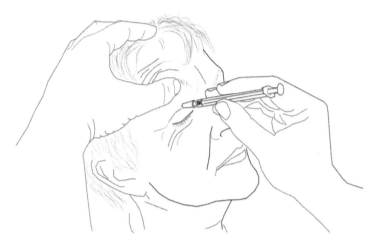

FIGURE PS15.2 Pass the needle just above the skin crease in the central lid

Apply corneal glue

CODE: PS16
TARGET YEAR OF ACHIEVEMENT: 7
AIM: to properly apply corneal glue to protect the eye with a corneal perforation.

BACKGROUND
A corneal perforation may be a consequence of trauma, infection or inflammation. Adequately closing the leak is important to reduce the risk of intraocular infection. Gluing may also help to control the progress of inflammatory corneal melt.

Either cyanoacrylate or fibrin glues may be used.

CONSENT
- Purpose: to seal the leaking wound.
- Serious or commonly occurring complications: infection, scarring, reduced vision, post-operative discomfort, need for drops after procedure.

EQUIPMENT LIST
- Glue (cyanoacrylate or fibrin)
- Chloramphenicol ointment
- Plastic drape
- Biopsy punch
- Sterile cotton bud
- Ocular sticks or eye spears
- Bandage contact lens

PROCEDURE
1 Prepare the adnexa, drape the patient and, if the patient is likely to move or squeeze their lids, place a lid speculum.
2 Cut a circular disc from the drape using the biopsy punch.
3 Dry the corneal surface around the defect.
4 Place a coil of chloramphenicol ointment on the cotton bud.
5 Pick up the disc using the cotton bud, then apply glue to the other side of the disc.
6 Invert the disc onto the dried corneal surface over the defect, glue side down.
7 Press the disc onto the surface lightly, and hold it in place while the glue sets.
8 Remove the cotton bud, leaving the disc glued in place, with ointment over the top.
9 Apply a bandage contact lens (*see* PS14, p. 80).
   ➤ The plastic disc will remain in place under the bandage contact lens and may remain there until the defect has closed or more definitive measures are required.

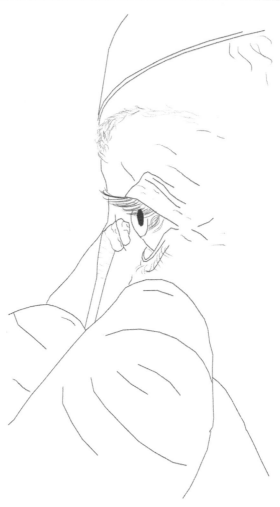

FIGURE PS16 Firmly distract the lower lid, and place the glue onto the cornea using the cotton bud

Perform anterior-chamber sampling

CODE: PS19
TARGET YEAR OF ACHIEVEMENT: 7
AIM: to obtain a sample of aqueous for microbiological or cytological investigation.

BACKGROUND
The most common scenario for aqueous sampling is in endophthalmitis, in which the bacteriological identification of the pathogen directs management. Cytological assessment may be appropriate in some intraocular tumours (retinoblastoma) and certain cases of uveitis.

EQUIPMENT LIST
- Topical anaesthesia
- Povidone iodine (5%)
- Insulin syringe with barrel removed

CONSENT
- Purpose: to obtain a microbiological/cytological diagnosis to direct management.
- Serious or commonly occurring complications: pain, infection, hypotony, damage to ocular structures including the iris and lens causing loss or reduction in vision, negative sample.

PROCEDURE
Before undertaking this procedure, it is sensible to discuss the case with microbiology, which will advise on its preferred transport medium and volume of sample.
1 Ensure patient comfort at the slit lamp.
2 Instil topical anaesthesia and povidone iodine.
3 Stabilise the needle tip (with the bevel away from the globe) on the temporal limbal cornea then firmly advance into the anterior chamber, ensuring a long intrastromal tract parallel to the plane of the iris.
4 As the needle tip enters the anterior chamber, the resistance will reduce. If the tip is not parallel to the iris plane, it may damage the anterior capsule of the phakic patient or disturb the IOL in the pseudophake.
5 The needle should stay within the anterior chamber. Observe droplets of aqueous passing into the barrel of the syringe.
6 Remove the needle along the same track and sheath or fit a stopper to the syringe.
7 Instil antibiotic drops and lightly pad the eye.

CODE: PS22
TARGET YEAR OF ACHIEVEMENT: 1
AIM: to irrigate ocular contaminants in an emergency setting and to be able to assess and interpret ocular-surface pH in this context.

BACKGROUND

Corneal and conjunctival contamination by environmental and industrial chemicals carries significant morbidity. Prompt removal of the offending agent and recognition of the important prognostic factors are a key skill for the trainee. Alkaline burns have the gravest prognosis, and, after establishing a high forniceal pH, irrigation should not be delayed. After the irrigation is started, it is important to ask if the contaminating agent was in liquid or powder form. Dry powder agents (such as lime and cement dust) easily become caked in the superior fornix, resisting attempts to irrigate them out – therefore, if the pH remains high in these patients despite irrigation, it is essential to double evert the lids and manually remove any powder residue.

EQUIPMENT LIST

- Topical anaesthesia
- Irrigating solution (NaCl [0.9%] or balanced salt solution)
- Intravenous (IV) giving set
- Morgan® Lens
- Desmarres retractor
- Litmus paper
- Cotton bud

PROCEDURE

Irrigation of the fornix may be undertaken using the Morgan Lens or an IV giving set. The Morgan Lens should not be used if there is suspicion of penetrating or perforating injury.

1 Instil adequate topical anaesthesia.
2 Bend back the tip of a strip of litmus paper, and place this over the lower lid margin into the inferior fornix. Compare the colour reaction with the key to establish the pH.
3 Place the Morgan Lens on the ocular surface or give the tip of the IV giving set to the patient to hold within the palpebral aperture and run through at least 1 L of irrigating fluid.
4 Recheck the pH after irrigation has finished. Continue to irrigate until the pH remains normalised.
5 If the pH remains high, double evert the lid to remove caked dry powder using the Desmarres retractor:
   a place the lip of the retractor in the superior lid sulcus with the handle down, then hold the lid margin against the shaft of the retractor and gently reflect handle upwards to evert lid
   b remove any caked material with a cotton bud.

Forced-duction testing

CODE: PS24
TARGET YEAR OF ACHIEVEMENT: 7
AIM: to differentiate between mechanical and paretic limitation of ocular movement.

BACKGROUND

When planning strabismus surgery, if the action of a muscle appears reduced, it is important to rule out the presence of a paretic component. The forced-duction and force-generation tests differentiate paretic from mechanical restriction and are usually carried out in theatre.

EQUIPMENT LIST

- Topical anaesthesia
- Notched forceps

It is wise to undertake a forced duction test before any strabismus surgery. The patient is usually under general anaesthesia before the test is undertaken as it is uncomfortable and unnecessary to undertake outside of this context.

Force generation testing can only be undertaken on a conscious patient; it is very important therefore to establish excellent topical anaesthesia prior to testing.

PROCEDURE

Forced-duction test

1 Grasp the limbus lightly with the forceps.
  ➤ This is most easily done by gently retropulsing the globe 2–3 mm with open forceps at the surgical limbus, then closing the forceps to hold the conjunctiva, before relaxing the retropulsion.
2 Ask the patient to look in the direction of gaze to be tested.
3 Rotate the globe gently towards the direction of gaze being tested, taking care to rotate around the Z-axis (the centre of rotation of the globe) and without retropulsing the globe in the socket.
  ➤ In paretic limitation, the globe will move freely with assistance (passive duction).
  ➤ When a mechanical restriction is present, the passive movement will be stiff and perhaps incomplete.

Force-generation test

- Direct the patient to look away from the field of action of the muscle being tested.
- Grasp the limbus as detailed in Step 1 of the 'Forced-duction test', and ask the patient to look slowly to the direction being tested.
  ➤ The force of the duction will be felt, allowing for a more objective assessment.
  ➤ In normal subjects, the speed of duction will be sufficient to tear the conjunctiva – be prepared to let go.

Surgical skills

Surgical measures for protection of the ocular surface

CODE: SS8

TARGET YEAR OF ACHIEVEMENT: 7

AIM: to establish temporary or permanent protection of the ocular surface to encourage the re-epithelialisation of chronic corneal ulcers.

CLINICAL CONTEXT

Lid malposition – in particular, entropion – and lash mid-direction are an important cause of corneal co-morbidity. Bedside repositioning of the lid is an important step in the treatment of corneal ulcers in the context of entropion.

There are many options available for the surgical protection of the ocular surface; the methods described here are two of the most common and practical options. However, the most appropriate solution in any particular case is tailored to that case and local guidance.

EVERTING SUTURES

Everting sutures are a simple and straightforward technique used to improve the lid position and reduce traumatic corneal injury to allow healing. The sutures plicate and redirect the pull of the lower-lid retractors to the anterior tarsal surface, stabilising the lid.

Equipment list

- Lignocaine (2%) with 1:80 000 adrenaline
- Three double-armed 5/0 Vicryl® sutures on cutting needles
- Adson, Lister or St Martins forceps and needle holders

Anatomical landmark

- The lower-lid retractors are found in the inferior fornix as a white linear band deep to the forniceal conjunctiva.

Procedure

1 Anaesthetise the lid margin, tarsus and tarsal conjunctiva.
2 Grasp the lid margin with toothed forceps, and reflect downwards as the patient looks up, identifying the retractors in the fornix (a white band, deep within the fornix).
3 Engage the retractors with the needle tip, and pass the needle through the lid, towards the lid margin, emerging just anterior to the lash line.
4 The second arm should be placed adjacent to the first, as a horizontal mattress.
5 Place two or three such sutures, evenly spaced along the lid, taking care not to injure the canaliculus medially.
6 Tie each suture, starting laterally, so that the lid margin is just everted.
7 Check the extent of retractor plication by asking the patient to look down – the lower lid should move down with this movement.

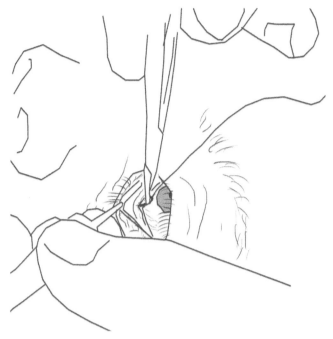

FIGURE SS8.1 Identify position of lower lid retractors

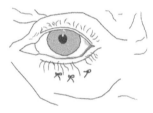

FIGURE SS8.2 Position of everting sutures

TARSORRHAPHY
Clinical context
Neurotrophic and chronic non-healing ulcers, especially those exacerbated by lagophthalmos – as seen in facial-nerve palsy and thyroid eye disease – may require permanent or semi-permanent closure of the lid to protect the ocular surface and to promote healing.

Sutured temporary tarsorrhaphy
Equipment list
- Lignocaine (2%) with 1:80 000 adrenaline and syringe with grey needle
- Double-armed 4/0 nylon suture with a cutting needle
- Narrow gauge silicone tubing (as found on a butterfly cannula), cut into two lengths of around 10 mm each as bolsters
- Antibiotic ointment

Anatomical landmark
- The anterior and posterior lamellae of the lid meet at the grey line – the sutures should pass through this landmark.

Procedure

1 Infiltrate the upper and lower lid and lid margin with local anaesthetic.
2 Place the suture through one of the silicone tube bolster segments.
3 For the lower-lid suture, enter the lid at around 5 mm inferior to the lid margin, pass through the tarsal plate then exit the lower lid through the grey line.
4 Follow the same tract with the other arm but with a more lateral position.
5 The upper-lid suture should mirror the path of the lower-lid suture, entering through the grey line and exiting 5 mm below the lash line.
6 Pass the second bolster through, and tie the suture with a releasable knot.
7 Apply antibiotic ointment to the sutures.

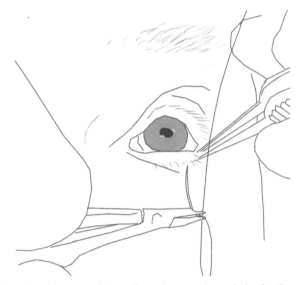

FIGURE SS8.3 Enter the skin around 5 mm from the margin and aim for the grey line

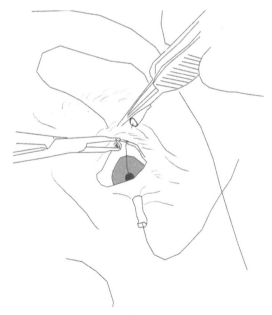

FIGURE SS8.4 Pass suture through the grey line

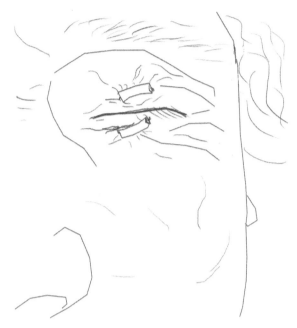

FIGURE SS8.5 Closed lid with bolsters in place

> **Pearls**
> ▶ The bolsters prevent suture damage to the skin and encourage eversion of the lashes to prevent trichiatic corneal abrasion.
> ▶ Releasable sutures are favoured to facilitate prompt reversal and ease of examination.
> ▶ To avoid them rubbing against the ocular surface, sutures should not pass posterior to the grey line.
> ▶ A temporary tarsorrhaphy may be performed in clinic or at the bedside.

Permanent three-layer tarsorrhaphy
Equipment list
- Lignocaine (2%) with 1:80 000 adrenaline and syringe with grey needle
- Number 15 blade
- Westcott scissors
- Bipolar cautery
- Absorbable suture (5/0) on a double-armed quarter-circle cutting needle
- Suture (6/0) for skin (surgeon's preference)

Consent
- Purpose: to provide permanent protection to the ocular surface when visual rehabilitation is not expected.
- Serious or commonly occurring complications: infection, irreversible lid closure, poor cosmesis.

Procedure
1 Infiltrate the lids and lid margin with local anaesthetic.
2 Perform a grey-line split and dissect the tarsus from the orbicularis and skin, forming a muscle/skin flap, and mobilise the tarsus.

3 Further dissect the muscle/skin flap into separate layers consisting of the orbicularis and skin.

4 Appose the upper- and lower-lid tarsus with the 5/0 absorbable suture, being careful to take partial thickness bites.

5 Close the muscle layer with the 6/0 absorbable suture then close the skin – ensuring the lashes are externalised at the palpebral aperture.

Pearls

▶ To avoid abrading the ocular surface, the tarsal sutures must not pass through the tarsal conjunctival surface.

▶ The extent of lid closure can be tailored to the particular case. Generally, a lateral position will allow for the instillation of drops and examination of the eye while affording improved protection.

CODE: SS9
TARGET YEAR OF ACHIEVEMENT: 7
AIM: to release the lateral canthal tendon to relieve intra-orbital pressure in retrobulbar haemorrhage.

CLINICAL CONTEXT

Traumatic retrobulbar haemorrhage may cause significant elevation in intra-orbital pressure leading to optic nerve ischaemia. The eyelids prevent anterior displacement of the globe to relieve this pressure leading to further ischaemia. Where intra-orbital pressure is elevated due to retrobulbar haemorrhage the globe may be mobilised by surgically releasing the lateral canthal tendons.

EQUIPMENT LIST

- Local anaesthesia with adrenaline
- Straight sharp scissors
- Artery clip
- Toothed forceps
- Bipolar cautery

CONSENT

- Purpose: to decompress the orbit and prevent blindness and/or loss of the eye.
- Serious or commonly occurring complications: bleeding, scars, need for reconstruction, damage to extraocular muscles causing squint/diplopia.

ANATOMICAL LANDMARKS

- The lateral canthal tendon arises at the lateral orbital rim and divides into superior and inferior limbs at the lateral canthal angle.
- The inferior tarsal plate is approximately 5 mm deep and is formed by fibres continuous with the tendon.

PROCEDURE

1 Clean the lids and temporal skin.
2 Inject local anaesthetic along both limbs of the tendon and into the deep tissues posterior to the lateral canthal angle.
3 Open the jaws of the artery clip and place one deep into the inferior fornix at the lateral angle, aiming to grasp the inferior canthal tendon close to its insertion.
4 Close tightly for 20–30 seconds to devascularise the surgical field.
5 Remove the artery clip and place the open blades of the scissors in the same position.
6 Make a cut through the inferior tendon whilst stabilising the lid margin with forceps
7 Distract the lid inferiorly with the forceps to check that the tendon is fully released.
8 Reassess the pressure in the orbit – if it remains elevated, ensure that the inferior tendon is fully divided. Rarely, consider the same procedure for the superior canthal tendon.
9 The cut ends can be cauterised to prevent post-operative bleeding.
10 Reassess orbital pressure and optic nerve function.
11 After the orbit is decompressed, place a single pad, without pressure, over the eye.

> **Pearl**
> ▶ It is important to check and document optic-nerve function (particularly for RAPD and VA) prior to this procedure.

POST-OPERATIVE CONSIDERATION

● The lateral canthal tendons may be reconstructed as a secondary procedure or left to heal by secondary intention – persistent laxity following this procedure may result in lid malposition.

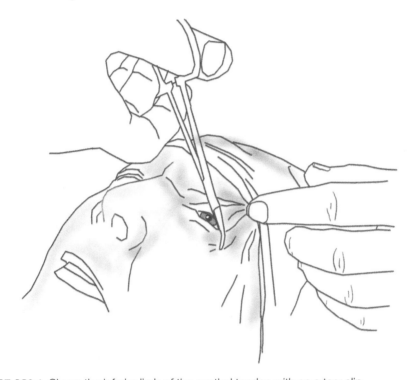

FIGURE SS9.1 Clamp the inferior limb of the canthal tendon with an artery clip

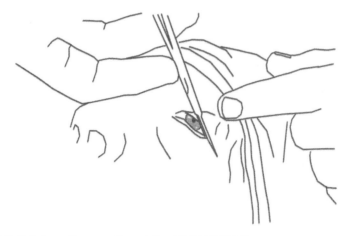

FIGURE SS9.2 Cut down the same line as the clamped tissue

CODE: SS10
TARGET YEAR OF ACHIEVEMENT: 7
AIM: to establish histological diagnosis of lid lesions.

LID BIOPSIES

Equipment list
- Local anaesthesia with adrenaline
- Lid tray
- Gentian violet sterile skin marker
- Number 15 blade or cutting cautery
- Suture (6/0) for skin closure
- Antibiotic ointment

Consent
- Purpose: for diagnosis and treatment.
- Serious or commonly occurring complications: scars, infection, further surgery, incomplete margins.

Surgical options
- To maximise the chances of a positive biopsy and acceptable wound healing, the surgeon must decide on the correct approach to the lesion. For discrete lesions of the lid and adnexal skin, it is usually appropriate to perform an excision biopsy with adequate margins. For morphoeic lesions or when the diagnosis may be in question, it may be appropriate to perform an incisional biopsy to confirm the diagnosis before planning more extensive surgery.
- Horizontal incisions on the lid should be avoided, as their reconstruction is likely to induce ectropion.
- Simple excisions of discrete lesions may be closed at the same time as biopsy. In cases in which the margins are uncertain, it may be advisable to plan for delayed closure until after histological confirmation of complete excision.

Procedure
1 Measure and mark either the excision margins around the lesion or the planned orientation of the incisions.
2 Check that the position of the planned incisions will allow for adequate reconstruction – if not, consider more complex reconstructive techniques, including free flaps, pedicle grafts and sliding flaps.
3 Incise to the full thickness of the skin, ensuring uniformity around the lesions.
4 Having made the incisions as per the skin markings, pick up one apex and dissect away from the subcutaneous tissue with scissors, using the full length of the blade, if possible.
5 Maintain orientation of the biopsy lesion by placing non-absorbable sutures at various points on the sampled tissue, referring to these on the histology form.
6 Establish haemostasis.
7 Reconstruct the wound or leave it for staged closure.
8 Apply antibiotic ointment and pad.

Pearl

▶ The skin of the lid is significantly thinner and more fragile than that of the brow. This is particularly true in older patients and must be borne in mind when executing incisions involving this boundary.

CODE: SS11
TARGET YEAR OF ACHIEVEMENT: 7
AIM: to obtain sufficient vascular and perivascular tissue to allow histological assessment in cases of suspected giant-cell arteritis.

EQUIPMENT LIST
- Skin marker
- Local anaesthesia
- Sterile field
- Scalpel with number 15 blade and surgical tray including artery clips and cat's claw retractors
- Bipolar cautery
- Absorbable suture
- Skin suture
- Histology transport pot

CONSENT
- Purpose: to establish diagnosis of giant-cell arteritis.
- Serious or commonly occurring complications: stroke (extremely rare), scalp necrosis (extremely rare), pain during procedure, damage to facial nerve causing partial facial-nerve palsy, scarring, bruising, failure to obtain histological diagnosis.

ANATOMICAL LANDMARKS
- The external temporal artery arises within the parotid gland and may be palpated just anterior to the tragus.
- It bifurcates into frontal and parietal branches 5 cm above the zygoma. At this point, it lies deep to the auricularis anterior muscle and within the superficial temporal fascia.
- The temporal branch of the facial nerve (inv. frontalis) accompanies the artery within this fascial plane but extends anteriorly towards the brow, while the artery proceeds posteriorly over the ear.

PROCEDURE
1 Shave the skin in the territory of the temporal artery.
2 Mark the course of the artery – with or without Doppler guidance.
3 Prepare the surgical field and drape.
4 Make a full-thickness skin incision adjacent to the expected route of the artery, through subcutaneous fat.
5 Using blunt dissection with cautery explore the fascia until the artery is located
6 Directly palpate the pulse of the artery with a fingertip in the wound if it is difficult to find.
7 Identify the artery (see Figure SS11.2) and dissect the perivascular tissue at its distal and proximal ends such that an absorbable suture may be passed around the artery for ligation.
8 As at least 20 mm of the artery should be removed, ensure the ligatures are at least 25 mm apart to allow for a small stump to be left.
9 Firmly tie the ligature at the proximal end followed by the distal end.
10 Cut the artery within the ligatures and place in the histology transport pot.
11 Ensure haemostasis.
12 Close in layers.

POST-OPERATIVE CONSIDERATION

- In cases with a high clinical index of suspicion, steroid therapy should not be delayed until histological analysis is provided.

> **Pearls**
> - Giant-cell arteritis is characterised by 'skip lesions' – your biopsy may not yield a positive result even in 'classic disease'.
> - The sensitivity of temporal artery biopsy after a week's steroid therapy is significantly reduced – if possible, the procedure should precede medical therapy.
> - Check for steal syndrome before biopsy – with the patient seated upright, palpate the carotid and occlude against carotid buttress with firm pressure – if the patient develops dizziness or light headedness this may signify a steal syndrome, in this case, try the other side.
> - 'S'-shaped incisions allow for better exposure and longer artery harvest.

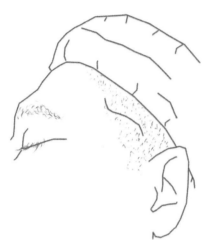

FIGURE SS11.1 Shave the skin and mark the artery prior to skin preparation

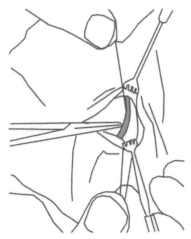

FIGURE SS11.2 Identify the artery and expose at least 20 mm before passing proximal and distal ligatures

CODE: SS14
TARGET YEAR OF ACHIEVEMENT: 3
AIM: to improve VA by displacing the opacified posterior capsule from the visual axis in a pseudophakic eye.

EQUIPMENT LIST
- Mydriatic agents
- YAG laser
- Capsulotomy contact lens (e.g. Abraham)
- Coupling agent
- Topical anaesthesia
- Ocular antihypertensive agent

LASER SETTINGS
- Offset: 1.50
- Power: 1.5–2.5 mW

CONSENT
- Purpose: to improve vision
- Serious or commonly occurring complications: reduced vision (IOL pits causing dysphotopsia, retinal burn/detachment, corneal burn), raised IOP, further procedures.

PROCEDURE
1 Dilate the patient's pupil.
2 Ensure patient and operator comfort at the laser.
3 Instil topical anaesthesia.
4 Place the contact lens and align the HeNe, aiming the beam at the posterior capsule.
5 Arm the laser and deliver single shots to the posterior capsule.
   ➤ The pattern of shots may be an incomplete circle (leave an intact bridge inferiorly) or across the visual axis (there is a higher risk of dysphotopsia if lens pits are created on the visual axis).
6 Continue the treatment until the posterior capsule falls away from the visual axis.
7 Ensure the laser is disarmed at the end of treatment.
8 Instil the ocular antihypertensive agent.

POST-OPERATIVE CONSIDERATIONS
- Warn patients of the symptoms of retinal detachment and raised IOP.
- Routine follow-up is not mandatory for straightforward capsulotomies.

Laser for management of raised intraocular pressure

CODE: SS15
TARGET YEAR OF ACHIEVEMENT: 3

YAG PERIPHERAL IRIDOTOMY

Aim: to provide alternative routes of aqueous flow from posterior to anterior chamber in cases of pupil block where the normal transpupillary pathways are compromised.

Equipment list
- YAG laser
- Topical anaesthesia
- Miotic agent
- Anterior-segment contact lens (Abraham, PI)
- Coupling agent
- Topical steroid
- Topical antihypertensive
- Pilocarpine (2%)

Laser settings
- Offset: 0.0–1.5 mm
- Power: 2.0–4.0 mJ (titrate to response)

Some clinicians advocate double shots in rapid sequence (set on the laser machine), as this can produce extra disruption for less power delivered.

Consent
- Purpose: to reduce the risk of pupil block and angle-closure glaucoma.
- Serious or commonly occurring complications: dysphotopsia, failure of treatment, further treatment, discomfort.

Procedure
1 Instil the miotic agent at least 15 minutes prior to the procedure (several drops over 15–20 minutes).
2 Ensure the laser settings are selected and that the laser is on standby.
3 Position the patient at the slit lamp after instillation of topical anaesthesia.
4 Place the lens on the cornea and orientate the magnifying portion superiorly.
5 If possible, identify iris crypts, and target these.
6 Arm the laser.
7 Align the HeNe aiming beams and discharge the laser.
8 Observe for a gush of pigment into the anterior chamber, which is a positive sign of complete iridotomy.
9 Ensure the laser is disarmed at the end of the treatment.

Post-operative consideration
- Iopidine (1%) immediately and steroid (0.1% dexamethasone) four times per day for 4 days.

> **Pearls**
> ▶ Dark irides can be resistant to YAG energy; these can be pretreated with single-spot argon burns prior to YAG iridotomy.
> ▶ Larger iridotomies tend to be more effective than smaller ones.
> ▶ Avoid placing the iridotomy within the tear film meniscus as this is likely to cause dysphotopsia. A position under the upper lid is preferable.

SELECTIVE LASER TRABECULOPLASTY
Aim: to increase aqueous drainage by opening the trabecular meshwork.

Equipment list
- Selective laser trabeculoplasty (SLT) laser
- SLT goniolens
- Topical anaesthesia
- Topical antihypertensives

Laser settings
- Power: 1.0 mJ
- Duration: 0.3 s
- Spot size: 400 µm

Consent
- Purpose: to reduce IOP.
- Serious or commonly occurring complications: mild discomfort.

Procedure
1 Instil antihypertensive drops at least 15 minutes prior to undertaking the procedure.
2 Ensure that the laser settings are appropriate and the laser is in standby mode.
3 Instil topical anaesthesia.
4 Position the patient at laser slit lamp and place the goniolens on the cornea, and orientate the image, ensuring a clear view of the pigmented trabecular meshwork.
5 Arm the laser.
6 Focus the HeNe aiming beam on the pigmented trabecular meshwork.
7 Deliver single shots to the pigmented meshwork – a small bubble should be created by each shot.
  ➤ Titrate the power to the lowest setting that creates a bubble.
  ➤ Treatment may be 180–360 degrees, depending on the case – document the area of treatment clearly.
8 Ensure the laser is disarmed at the end of treatment.
9 Instil topical antihypertensives after the procedure.

ARGON-LASER TRABECULOPLASTY
Argon-laser trabeculoplasty (ALT) follows the same procedure as SLT, but the burns are applied to the junction of the pigmented and non-pigmented meshwork.

CYCLODIODE LASER
Aim: to reduce IOP by limiting aqueous production by the ciliary body in eyes with a poor visual prognosis and painfully high pressure.

Equipment list
- Diode laser with K-probe
- Appropriate laser goggles

- Lid speculum
- Periocular anaesthesia (sub-conjunctival, sub-Tenon's or peribulbar)
- Transillumination probe or endoilluminator

Laser settings
- Power: 1000–2500 mW
- Duration: 1500–2000 ms

Consent
- Purpose: to produce a long-term reduction in IOP.
- Serious or commonly occurring complications: hypotony/hypertension, significant intraocular inflammation, further treatments, discomfort, hyphaema, reduced vision.

Procedure
1 Place the lid speculum and ensure adequate analgesia.
2 Confirm the position of the ciliary body by transilluminating the anterior segment – the transilluminating probe tip should be placed on or close to the surgical limbus; the outline of the insertion of the ciliary body is demonstrated by a shadow behind the limbus.
3 Place the heel of the K-probe at the limbus, so that the laser will deliver to the ciliary body (as located in Step 2).
4 Deliver the laser burns.
   ➤ The power may be titrated until a pop sound is heard on applying the laser. Reduce power slightly at this point.
5 Ensure the laser is disarmed at the end of treatment.

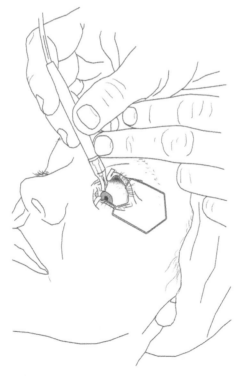

FIGURE SS15 Cyclodiode laser. To deliver effective treatment, the probe must be flat against the globe

Post-operative considerations

- Place between 20 and 30 evenly spaced burns per 180 degrees.
- Avoid the 3 and 9 o'clock positions (insertions of the ciliary nerves).
- Diode laser often induces a profound fibrinous uveitis – patients should be given intensive topical steroids, and periocular depot steroid may be considered.

Laser for retinal disease

BACKGROUND
The proper application of a retinal laser takes years to master. In part, this is because it takes this period of time to follow up patients and observe the effect of their treatment. For this reason, didactic instruction on settings, patterns of burns and frequency of application is not appropriate. The clinician should understand why the laser is required, how the treatment works and what they are expecting to achieve.

Laser settings
The energy delivered is dependent on the energy developed by the laser, the length of the burn and the spot size. In turn, the spot size is altered by the magnification of the lens; clinicians should be aware of the magnifying effect of each of the lenses they use. Energy absorption is primarily affected by RPE pigmentation; therefore, a myopic blonde fundus reflects much of the incident energy, thus requires higher power settings than a highly pigmented fundus.

Photocoagulation laser
The advent of the Pascal™ Photocoagulator (Topcon, United States) patterned-scanning laser has allowed the delivery of photocoagulation laser to the retina in near simultaneously delivered grids of up to 25 burns. This significantly reduces the time taken to undertake retinal laser treatment, as well as allowing greater reproducibility between clinicians. Settings for Pascal laser use are typically greater than for single-shot argon or frequency-doubled neodymium-doped yttrium aluminium garnet (Nd:YAG) systems. In every case, it is essential to titrate burns to the response and to adjust these across the retina as absorption patterns change. Modern photocoagulating laser burns do not spread over time, as was the case with older systems such as the xenon arc laser. This makes protection of peripheral fields – in particular, the driving field – more predictable. Nonetheless, it is important to explain to the patient the potential for loss of field prior to undertaking laser treatment. If posterior pole laser treatment is undertaken, the patient should be counselled on the risk to the driving field.

It is important to bear in mind that photocoagulation is a destructive intervention, in particular, with young patients and those who rely on driving for their livelihood. In practical terms, this means avoiding applying pan-retinal photocoagulation (PRP)

TABLE SS16

Lens	Spot-size magnification factor
Volk Area Centralis®	0.94
Volk QuadrAspheric®	1.97
Volk SuperQuad®	2.00
Ocular® Mainster	1.03
Ocular Mainster Wide Field	0.73
Ocular Mainster PRP	0.57
Ocular Mainster High Magnification	1.34

within 3 disc diameters (DD) of the nasal disc margin and 3 DD temporal to the fovea. PRP can be delivered up to the outer edges of the arcades without threatening the driving field *in most cases.*

SLIT LAMP–DELIVERED PAN-RETINAL PHOTOCOAGULATION

Aim: to induce regression of neovascular retinopathy and to prevent its development in the presence of marked retinal ischaemia by reducing the retinal oxygen tension.

Equipment list
- Laser (514 nm, argon green, frequency-doubled YAG [potassium titanyl phosphate {KTP}])
- Wide-angle contact lens with anti-reflective coating (e.g. QuadrAspheric®, Mainster PRP, SuperQuad®)
- Topical mydriatics
- Topical anaesthesia
- Coupling fluid

Consent
- Purpose: to halt/reverse new vessel disease.
- Serious or commonly occurring complications: reduction of peripheral field (potential implication for driving licence), symptomatic scotoma, discomfort, reduced night vision, reduced colour vision, need for further laser treatment.

Procedure
1 Instil topical mydriatics and topical anaesthetic.
2 Confirm the laser settings, and position the patient at the laser slit lamp.
3 Place the lens on the cornea with coupling fluid.
4 Confirm the location of the disc, fovea and macula.
5 Arm the laser.
6 Titrate single burns in the peripheral retina until light burns are seen.
7 Delineate the limit of the intended treatment with a single ring of burns.
   ➤ All treatment thereafter should be delivered peripheral to this line to reduce the risk of inadvertently straying into the posterior pole and applying macular burns.
8 Deliver between 1000 and 1500 burns in the initial treatment sessions, spacing the burns 1.5–2.0 burn-widths apart.
   ➤ To preserve the driving field, avoid the macula and the area nasal to the disc equivalent to 3 DD. Burns may be applied up to the temporal watershed zone (approximately 3 DD temporal to the fovea).
   ➤ Burns can safely be delivered up to the vascular arcades, although treatment should start peripherally.
9 Ensure the laser is disarmed at the end of treatment.

Pearls
▹ The advent of the Pascal laser has significantly reduced the time spent at the slit lamp, for both patient and clinician. Using this system, grids of varying size and number of burns can be delivered in a short space of time. Pascal burns tend to be lighter than those delivered by a single-shot system – the importance of titration to each specific case, rather than using the same settings for all, must be underlined.
▹ The spot size on the retina should be around 500 μm – refer to the magnification factor for the lens being used.
▹ Treatment efficacy is dictated by the area of retinal coverage, not the number of burns – therefore, more burns are required if smaller spot sizes are used.

▶ In pre-proliferative or mild neovascular disease, peripheral PRP may be all that is required. Aggressive neovascularisation may require treatment up to the arcades.
▶ Loss of driving field is very rare if the laser is applied properly.
▶ It is sensible to reorientate yourself from time to time to prevent inadvertently straying into the macula.

MACULAR ARGON-LASER PHOTOCOAGULATION: MACULAR GRID LASER

With the advent of intravitreal therapies – both anti-vascular endothelial growth factor (VEGF) and slow-release steroid preparations – use of macular laser is declining. Nonetheless, it remains an important tool, particularly in cases of eccentric or recalcitrant macular oedema. The chances of macular laser causing a symptomatic scotoma are much higher than a pan-retinal laser, and this should be clearly discussed and documented prior to the procedure.

Spot sizes, energy levels, burn duration and number are all fewer/less than for any other retinal laser. Local policies and preferred practice should be followed, and the first macular laser applications undertaken by the trainee must be supervised by an experienced clinician.

Aim: to directly treat areas of clinically significant macular oedema (CSMO), as defined by the Early Treatment Diabetic Retinopathy Study (ETDRS) (*see* Appendix).

Equipment list
- Laser (514 nm, argon green, frequency-doubled YAG [KTP])
- High-magnification contact lens with anti-reflective coating (e.g. Area Centralis)
- Topical mydriatics
- Topical anaesthesia
- Coupling fluid

Consent
- Purpose: to stabilise vision.
- Serious or commonly occurring complications: symptomatic scotoma, vision may not improve, need for further procedures.

Procedure
1 Instil the topical mydriatics and topical anaesthetic.
2 Confirm the laser settings, and position the patient at the laser slit lamp.
3 Place the lens on the cornea with coupling fluid, and confirm the retinal anatomy.
4 Provide a target for the patient to look at – check that the patient is able to do this before applying burns.
5 Identify the fixation point by asking the patient to look at the slit beam with the laser in safe mode.
6 Arm the laser.
7 Titrate single burns in the extra-macular retina – titrate the power until the burn is just visible on the retina then reduce the power until the burn is not visible before treating within the macula (some practitioners advocate a burn that is just visible after 2–3 seconds).
8 Treat the target area using a grid or modified grid pattern, with burns around two spot diameters apart.
9 Ensure the burns remain at an equal level, bearing in mind that power may need to be increased in areas of significant oedema.
10 Ensure the laser is disarmed at the end of treatment.

Pearls

▶ The Pascal laser may be used, with caution, for macular laser. The potential for causing permanent central visual loss exists with this laser, and so it should not be used until the clinician is comfortable with it.

▶ Focal laser may be delivered, using similar settings, as individual burns to discrete lesions of leakage associated with micro-aneurysms.

▶ Clearly identify the fixation point, bearing in mind that *fixation may not be foveal – particularly in vitrectomised and previously lasered eyes*.

▶ Do not treat fixation point or any area within the FAZ.

▶ Be cautious when applying burns within 100 µm of the FAZ, as they may mature over time, causing a symptomatic central scotoma.

▶ The treatment of central fluid with laser is probably outmoded in the era of intra-vitreal therapies.

ARGON-LASER RETINOPEXY

Aim: to secure the neurosensory retina to the RPE in areas of retinal tears and weakness.

Equipment list

- Laser (514 nm, argon green, frequency-doubled YAG [KTP])
- Wide-angle contact lens with anti-reflective coating (e.g. QuadrAspheric, Mainster PRP, SuperQuad)
- Topical mydriatics
- Topical anaesthesia
- Coupling fluid

Consent

- Purpose: to reduce the risk of retinal detachment.
- Serious or commonly occurring complications: symptomatic scotoma, discomfort, failure of treatment requiring surgical intervention.

Procedure

1 Instil the topical mydriatics and topical anaesthetic.
2 Confirm the laser settings, and position the patient at the laser slit lamp.
3 Place the lens on the cornea with coupling fluid, and confirm the retinal anatomy.
4 Provide a target for the patient to look at – confirm that the patient is able to do this before delivering burns.
5 Arm the laser.
6 Titrate single burns in the peripheral retina – aim for small white burns.
7 Encircle the target lesion with at least three concentric rings of burns.
8 Space the burns at one spot size apart, offsetting each row to cover the spaces in the previous row and overlapping the rows.
9 Ensure the anterior lip of the defect is encircled.
10 Ensure the laser is disarmed at the end of treatment.

Pearls

▶ The Pascal laser may be used for retinopexy using curve pattern presets.
▶ The indirect laser may be used with indentation to ensure anterior encirclement.

Appendix:
key studies and
guidelines

Fifty shades of grey: major eye studies of interest to ophthalmic trainees

Gwyn Samuel Williams

SECTION 1: GLAUCOMA

1 OHTS: Ocular Hypertension Treatment Study (2002)

Aim: to examine risk factors for the conversion of ocular hypertension (OHT) into primary open-angle glaucoma (POAG).

Details: 5-year follow-up, 1636 participants. Two groups: treated and observed. In the observed group, the aim was to both reduce IOP by 20% and reach 24 mmHg or less.

Outcome: *4.4% of those in the treated group, versus 9.5% in the control group, progressed* to POAG, with increased age, thinner central corneal thickness (CCT) and male sex being identified as risk factors.

2 EMGT: Early Manifest Glaucoma Trial (2002)

Aim: to compare the progression of patients with a known diagnosis of POAG with or without treatment and to examine factors influencing progression.

Details: 6-year follow-up, 255 participants. Two main arms: treated and observed. Treatment consisted of ALT with or without Xalatan® (latanoprost).

Outcome: disease progression was seen in 45% of the treated group and 62% of the untreated group, with *each 1 mmHg reduction in IOP accounting for a 10% less chance of progressing.*

3 CIGTS: Collaborative Initial Glaucoma Treatment Study (2001)

Aim: to compare medical therapy against surgical trabeculectomy in those with open-angle glaucoma.

Details: 5-year follow-up, 607 participants. Two main groups: surgical and medical (unspecified).

Outcome: surgery achieved a 48% mean reduction in IOP while a 35% reduction was achieved in the medical group, though there was *no significant difference in field loss.* There was a threefold increased risk of cataracts in the surgical group.

4 CNTGS: Collaborative Normal Tension Glaucoma Study (1998)

Aim: to determine whether treating normal-tension glaucoma results in less disease progression.

Details: 5-year follow-up, 140 participants. Two arms: untreated and treated. An IOP reduction of 30% was aimed for by medical or surgical means in the treated group.

Outcome: *treatment decreased progression*, as 12% of the treated patients progressed versus 35% of the untreated, though there was a high rate of cataract seen in the treated group.

5 AGIS: Advanced Glaucoma Intervention Study (2000)

Aim: to compare ALT with surgical trabeculectomy in treating patients with known POAG for whom medical therapy had failed.

Details: 7-year follow-up, 789 eyes of 591 participants. Two arms: ALT and trabeculectomy, with the other procedure performed if IOP was greater than 18 mmHg.

Outcome: if the *IOP was consistently less than 18 mmHg, there was no progression* in either group, though white patients did better with trabeculectomy first and black patients did better with ALT first.

6 GLTFS: Glaucoma Laser Trial Follow-up Study (1995)

Aim: to determine if there is a difference in IOP control and disease progression between patients treated with ALT and those treated with topical medication (pre-carbonic anhydrase inhibitors and prostaglandins).

Details: 7-year follow-up, 203 participants. Two arms: initial treatment with ALT and topical medication.

Outcome: initial treatment with *ALT was at least as effective as topical medication.*

7 FFSS: Fluorouracil Filtering Surgery Study (1996)

Aim: to determine if the addition of the antimetabolite 5FU (fluorouracil) to trabeculectomy procedures influences outcomes.

Details: 5-year follow-up, 213 participants. Two arms: trabeculectomy alone and trabeculectomy with post-operative 5FU injections.

Outcome: 51% of operations in the 5FU group versus 74% of those in the trabeculectomy-alone group were classified as failures. Although the *addition of 5FU increased the success rate*, there was a higher incidence of late-onset bleb leaks (9% vs 2%).

8 TVTS: Tube Versus Trabeculectomy Study (2012)

Aim: to compare success rates and complications between patients treated with the Baerveldt® glaucoma implant and Mitomycin C enhanced surgical trabeculectomy.

Details: 5-year follow-up, 212 participants. Two arms: randomisation to drainage implant or surgical trabeculectomy. All patients were pseudophakes.

Outcome: *tubes were associated with a lower failure rate* (29.8%), while the trabeculectomy failure rate was 46.9%, mostly due to the need to redo surgery. Long-term VA and IOP outcomes were similar.

SECTION 2: AGE-RELATED MACULAR DEGENERATION
1 TAP: Treatment of Age-related macular degeneration with Photodynamic therapy (2001)

Aim: to determine whether photodynamic therapy (PDT) is useful in treating classic neovascular age-related macular degeneration (nAMD).

Details: 2-year follow-up, 529 participants. Two arms: verteporfin PDT and placebo – applied if FFA showed evidence of leakage. Three-monthly follow-ups with FFA at each visit.

Outcome: *PDT patients were less likely to lose vision* (47% with more than 15 letters lost) versus those in the control group (62%), but this trend was only significant for predominantly classic lesions.

2 VIP: Verteporfin in Photodynamic Therapy (2001)

Aim: to determine whether PDT has any beneficial effect for patients with purely occult nAMD.

Details: 2-year follow-up, 307 participants. Two arms: verteporfin PDT and placebo – applied if FFA showed evidence of leakage. Three-monthly follow-ups with FFA at each visit.

Outcome: *PDT patients were less likely to lose vision* (54% with more than 15 letters lost) versus those in the control group (67%), and patients with smaller lesions and worse VA fared better.

3 ANCHOR: ANti vascular endothelial growth factor antibody for the treatment of predominantly classic CHORoidal neovascularization in age-related macular degeneration (2009)

Aim: to compare intravitreal ranibizumab and PDT for the treatment of predominantly classic nAMD.

Details: 2-year follow-up, 423 participants. Three arms: (1) PDT with sham injection, (2) sham PDT with 0.3 mg ranibizumab and (3) sham PDT with 0.5 mg ranibizumab. FFA with or without PDT every 3 months but injections monthly.

Outcome: the *ranibizumab patients lost fewer letters* (90% lost fewer than 15 letters) versus PDT patients (65.7%) with 40% gaining more than 15 letters (vs 6.3% of the PDT group).

4 MARINA: Minimally classic/occult trial of the Anti-VEGF antibody Ranibizumab IN the treatment of neovascular Age related macular degeneration (2006)

Aim: to determine if intravitreal ranibizumab is useful in treating patients with minimally classic or occult lesions previously not licensed for treatment with PDT.

Details: 2-year follow-up, 716 patients. Three arms: (1) sham injection, (2) 0.3 mg ranibizumab and (3) 0.5 mg ranibizumab.

Outcome: at 12 months, the *ranibizumab patients had lost less vision* (95% lost fewer than 15 letters) than those receiving sham (62%), while the ranibizumab patients were also more likely to gain vision (34% vs 5%).

5 SAILOR: Safety Assessment of Intravitreal Lucentis fOR AMD (2009)

Aim: to determine whether safety issues are involved in treating patients with ranibizumab and if there is a difference between the 0.3 mg and 0.5 mg doses.

Details: 1-year follow-up, 4300 participants. An amalgam of the MARINA and ANCHOR studies looking purely for safety signals.

Outcome: the *rate of serious ocular events was less than 1%*, with *no difference seen between the two doses* used.

6 PRONTO: The results of Variable Ranibizumab Dosing (2009)

Aim: to determine whether variable VA and OCT-guided ranibizumab therapy after three loading doses is comparable to ANCHOR and MARINA with regards visual outcomes.

Details: 2-year follow-up, 40 patients. A drop of five or more letters and/or an increase in OCT thickness of 100 μm or more resulted in an injection.

Outcome: the *VA outcomes were comparable to those obtained in the large studies*, with fewer injections required.

7 FOCUS: Ranibizumab combined with verteporfin photodynamic therapy in neovascular age-related macular degeneration (2008)

Aim: to determine if adding ranibizumab improves outcomes in patients receiving PDT.

Details: 2-year follow-up, 164 patients. Two arms: monthly intravitreal ranibizumab and monthly sham, with all patients receiving quarterly PDT as needed.

Outcome: *PDT with ranibizumab was more effective* than PDT alone, but results were worse than those obtained in ANCHOR and MARINA.

8 CATT: Comparison of Age-related macular degeneration Treatments Trials: Lucentis-Avastin (2012)

Aim: to compare ranibizumab with bevacizumab as well as monthly versus as-needed (*pro re nata* [PRN]) dosing for each of these drugs.

Details: 2-year follow-up, 1208 patients. Four study groups: (1) monthly administration of each drug for a year then re-randomised to (2) monthly or (3) PRN, and (4) PRN from the outset for each drug. A non-inferiority study in which five-letter differences were deemed non-inferior.

Outcome: *bevacizumab was non-inferior to ranibizumab*, as was PRN against monthly doses of the same drug. There was a higher adverse systemic event profile in the bevacizumab group (risk ratio 1.29).

9 AREDS 1: Age Related Eye Disease Study (2001)

Aim: to determine whether vitamins C and E, beta carotene and zinc have any effect on nAMD progression and VA.

Details: 6-year follow-up, 3640 participants. Four study groups: (1) zinc alone, (2) antioxidants alone, (3) zinc and antioxidants and (4) placebo.

Outcome: the *zinc plus antioxidant group experienced a 25% reduction in developing advanced AMD*. AREDS 2 (2013) showed lutein and zeaxanthin would be safer carotenoid supplements than the antioxidants of AREDS 1, although omega-3 fatty acids had no effect.

10 CABERNET: CNV secondary to AMD treated with Beta RadiatioN Epiretinal Therapy (2013)

Aim: to assess the safety and efficacy of epimacular brachytherapy as an additive treatment to PRN ranibizumab therapy for nAMD.

Details: 2-year follow-up, 494 participants. Two study groups: epimacular brachytherapy plus ranibizumab and ranibizumab alone.

Outcome: 77% of those in the epimacular brachytherapy group and 90% of those in the control group lost more than 15 letters; *the investigators do not support use of this technology*.

11 VIEW: VEGF trap-eye: Investigation of Efficacy and safety in Wet AMD (2012)

Aim: to see if aflibercept (VEGF trap eye) is equivalent in monthly and 2-monthly dosing regimens to monthly ranibizumab therapy.

Details: 2-year follow-up, 2419 patients. Four arms: (1) ranibizumab monthly, (2) aflibercept 0.5 mg monthly, (3) aflibercept 2 mg monthly and (4) aflibercept 2 mg every other month.

Outcome: intravitreal aflibercept at either monthly or every other month dosing was *equivalent to monthly ranibizumab therapy*.

12 EVEREST: Efficacy and safety of verteporfin photodynamic therapy in combination with ranibizumab or alone versus ranibizumab monotherapy in patients with symptomatic macular polypoidal choroidal vasculopathy (2012)

Aim: to determine if verteporfin PDT is better than 0.5 mg ranibizumab in treating the polypoidal choroidal vasculopathy variant of nAMD.

Details: 6-month follow-up, 61 patients. Three arms: (1) PDT plus sham ranibizumab, (2) sham PDT plus ranibizumab and (3) PDT plus ranibizumab.

Outcome: *PDT plus ranibizumab and PDT alone resulted in superior outcomes* in terms of the complete regression of polyps (77.8% and 71.4% vs 28.6%), although VA outcomes were not significantly different.

SECTION 3: NEURO-OPHTHALMOLOGY
1 ONTT: Optic Neuritis Treatment Trial (1999)

Aim: to examine the beneficial effects of corticosteroids in optic neuritis and the natural history of the disease.

Details: 15-year follow-up, 448 participants. Three arms: (1) oral prednisolone, (3) IV methylprednisolone and (3) oral placebo.

Outcome: 15-year follow-up demonstrated 25% risk of multiple sclerosis (MS) if magnetic resonance imaging (MRI) was normal at baseline and a 72% risk of MS if the MRI showed more than one white-matter lesion on MRI, whereas IV steroids resulted in quicker recovery but *no long-term decreased risk of MS*.

2 CHAMPS: Controlled High risk Avonex MultiPle Sclerosis study (2001)
Aim: to determine whether interferon beta-1a initiated at the time of a first episode of optic neuritis reduces the risk of definite conversion to clinical MS.
Details: 2-year follow-up, 192 participants. Two arms: patients treated with interferon beta-1a and those treated with placebo after the first episode of optic neuritis in patients demonstrating MRI evidence of subclinical demyelination.
Outcome: administration of *interferon beta-1a reduced the risk of development of clinically definite MS* in patients at high risk.

3 ETOMS: Early Treatment of Multiple Sclerosis study (2001)
Aim: to determine if interferon beta-1a initiated at the time of a first episode of optic neuritis reduces the risk of definite conversion to clinical MS in high-risk patients.
Details: 2-year follow-up, 308 participants. Two arms: study group of weekly subcutaneous interferon beta-1a for duration study and control group with placebo injections.
Outcome: *fewer patients converted to clinically definite MS in the interferon group* than in the placebo group (34% vs 45%, respectively).

4 NASCET: North American Symptomatic Carotid Endarterectomy Trial (1991)
Aim: to determine whether carotid endarterectomy reduces the risk of stroke in patients having had a transient ischaemic attack or a non-disabling stroke in the preceding 120 days.
Details: 2-year follow-up, 659 participants. Two arms: medical care and carotid endarterectomy surgery.
Outcome: *carotid endarterectomy reduced the risk of ipsilateral stroke* in symptomatic patients with stenosis of 70%–99% from 26% to 9% over the study period.

5 ACAS: Asymptomatic Carotid Atherosclerosis Study (1995)
Aim: to determine whether patients with asymptomatic carotid artery sclerosis greater than 60% benefit from carotid endarterectomy.
Details: 5-year follow-up, 1662 participants. Two arms: medical care and carotid endarterectomy surgery.
Outcome: *carotid endarterectomy reduced the risk of ipsilateral stroke* in asymptomatic patients from 11.0% to 5.1% over the study period.

SECTION 4: PAEDIATRICS
1 CRYO-ROP: Cryotherapy for Retinopathy of Prematurity (1990)
Aim: to ascertain if performing cryotherapy in pre-term babies with threshold retinopathy of prematurity (ROP) (defined as 5 contiguous or 8 non-contiguous hours of stage 3 ROP in zones 1 or 2 with plus disease) reduces unfavourable outcomes.
Details: 1-year follow-up, 291 participants. Two arms: cryotherapy and untreated.
Outcome: *cryotherapy was associated with fewer unfavourable fundal outcomes* (25.7% vs 47.4%) and improved VA results (unfavourable acuity in 35% vs 56.3%).

2 ETROP: Early Treatment of Retinopathy of Prematurity (2004)
Aim: to determine whether earlier treatment with laser retinal ablation of type 1 ROP (defined as stage 3 ROP or any stage ROP with plus disease in zone 1, or stage 2 or 3 *and* plus disease in zone 2) reduces unfavourable outcomes.
Details: 9-month follow-up, 317 participants. Participants had one eye randomised to early laser ablative treatment and the other to conventional therapy.
Outcome: *early treatment of type 1 ROP with laser ablation was associated with fewer unfavourable structural fundal outcomes* (9.0% vs 15.6%) and fewer unfavourable VA (14.3% vs 19.8%) results compared with conventional treatment.

3 BEAT-ROP: Bevacizumab Eliminates the Angiogenic Threat of Retinopathy Of Prematurity (2011)

Aim: to determine whether intravitreal bevacizumab is associated with reduced incidence of disease recurrence in babies with ROP stage 3 plus in zones 1 or 2.

Details: 1-year follow-up, 143 participants. Two groups: laser ablation therapy and intravitreal bevacizumab.

Outcome: *bevacizumab was associated with reduced recurrence of disease* in those with ROP in zone 1 but not those with ROP in zone 2.

SECTION 5: DIABETES

1 DCCT: Diabetes Control and Complications Trial (1993)

Aim: to determine whether intensive control of blood glucose reduces the rate of systemic complications in type 1 diabetics.

Details: 6-year follow-up, 1441 patients. Two groups: intensive glucose control with insulin pump or three or more daily injections, or conventional therapy with one or two daily injections.

Outcome: *intensive therapy reduced the development of diabetic retinopathy* by 76%, nephropathy by 54% and neuropathy by 60%.

2 UKPDS: United Kingdom Prospective Diabetes Study (1998)

Aim: to see if intensive control of blood glucose in newly diagnosed type 2 diabetics reduces the risk of systemic complications.

Details: 20-year follow-up, 3867 participants. Two groups: intensive treatment with insulin or a sulphonylurea and conventional, less intense therapy.

Outcome: with increased glucose control (HbA1c 7.0% vs 7.9%), there was a 21% *reduction in the progression of retinopathy*, with blood-pressure (BP) control also improving microvascular outcomes.

3 DRS: Diabetic Retinopathy Study (1976)

Aim: to determine the role of PRP in the evolution of proliferative diabetic retinopathy.

Details: 2-year follow-up, 1758 participants. All patients had one eye randomised to treatment (argon or xenon laser) and the other to no treatment.

Outcome: laser treatment with both modalities *reduced the incidence of severe visual loss by 50%.*

4 ETDRS: Early Treatment of Diabetic Retinopathy Study (1989)

Aim: to examine the natural history of diabetic retinopathy and the effects of various types of argon-laser treatment as well as *per os* (oral; p.o.) aspirin.

Details: 5-year follow-up, 3711 participants. Patients were divided into four groups: (1) p.o. aspirin or (2) p.o. placebo, and (3) laser treatment or (4) no laser treatment. Treated patients only had treatment in one eye which involved grid and scatter laser versus nothing in the control eye.

Outcome: aspirin demonstrated no clinically beneficial or harmful effects to the eyes. Grid laser was found *to decrease moderate visual loss in CSMO by 50%,* and guidelines defining timing of scatter laser as well as grading retinopathy were also developed.

5 DRVS: Diabetic Retinopathy Vitrectomy Study (1985)

Aim: to determine whether early vitrectomy affects outcomes in diabetics with a vitreous haemorrhage lasting at least 1 month and reducing vision to 6/300 or less.

Details: 2-year follow-up, 616 participants. Two arms: early vitrectomy and watchful waiting with a possibility of deferred vitrectomy.

Outcome: 25% of those in the early vitrectomy group had vision of 6/12 or better compared with 15% in the deferred group, with *younger type 1 diabetics with more severe proliferative diabetic retinopathy (PDR) benefitting the most* from vitrectomy.

6 BOLT: Bevacizumab Or Laser Treatment in managing diabetic macular edema (2012)

Aim: to compare intravitreal bevacizumab with argon macular laser in the treatment of CSMO associated with diabetic retinopathy.

Details: 2-year follow-up, 80 patients. Two arms: intravitreal bevacizumab and laser.

Outcome: *the bevacizumab group did better*, gaining a mean 8.6 ETDRS letters versus a mean loss of 0.5 letters in those undergoing macular laser therapy.

7 RESOLVE: Safety and efficacy of ranibizumab in diabetic macular edema (2010)

Aim: to ascertain if intravitreal ranibizumab is safe and effective in treating diabetic macular oedema.

Details: 1-year follow-up, 151 participants. Three arms: (1) 0.3 mg ranibizumab, (2) 0.5 mg ranibizumab, and (3) sham injection.

Outcome: *the ranibizumab groups did better*, with a mean gain of 10.3 letters in these groups versus a loss of 1.4 letters in the sham group. No safety concerns were raised.

8 READ-2: Two-year outcomes of the Ranibizumab for Edema of the mAcula in Diabetes (2010)

Aim: to determine whether laser, ranibizumab or both treatments together result in the best visual and structural outcomes in diabetic macular oedema.

Details: 2-year follow-up, 126 participants. Three arms: (1) ranibizumab, (2) laser and (3) combined laser and ranibizumab.

Outcome: *the patients receiving ranibizumab monotherapy did better*, gaining a mean of 7.4 letters, while the laser monotherapy group lost 0.5 letters and the combined group gained 3.8 letters.

9 RESTORE: Ranibizumab monotherapy or combined with laser versus laser monotherapy for diabetic macular edema (2011)

Aim: to determine whether laser, ranibizumab or both treatments together result in the best visual and structural outcomes in diabetic macular oedema.

Details: 1-year follow-up, 345 participants. Three groups: (1) ranibizumab plus sham laser, (2) sham injection plus laser and (3) ranibizumab plus laser.

Outcome: *the patients receiving ranibizumab monotherapy did better*, gaining a mean of 6.1 letters, while the laser monotherapy group gained 0.8 letters and the combined group gained 5.9 letters.

10 DRCR.net Protocol I: The Diabetic Retinopathy Clinical Research Network. Randomised trial evaluating ranibizumab plus prompt or deferred laser or triamcinolone plus prompt laser for diabetic macular edema (2010)

Aim: to compare ranibizumab, triamcinolone and laser treatments in patients with diabetic macular oedema.

Details: 1-year follow-up, 854 eyes of 691 participants. Four study groups: (1) sham injection plus laser, (2) ranibizumab plus laser, (3) triamcinolone plus laser and (4) ranibizumab plus deferred laser.

Outcome: *the two groups receiving ranibizumab had the best visual outcomes* and the laser plus sham group the worst. VA in the triamcinolone plus laser group was as good as ranibizumab in pseudophakic eyes but was associated with raised IOP.

11 FAME: Fluocinolone Acetonide for Macular Edema (2012)

Aim: to assess the efficacy and safety of sustained-release intravitreal fluocinolone implants (Iluvien®) in patients with diabetic macular oedema that is persisting despite previous laser therapy.

Details: 3-year follow-up, 953 participants. Three arms: (1) sham implant, (2) low-dose implant (0.2 µg/d) and (3) high-dose implant (0.5 µg/d).

Outcome: at 3 years, 28% of those receiving *high-dose implants reported a significantly increased rate of visual improvement* of more than 15 letters versus 19% in the sham group, though virtually all phakic patients developed cataract and 8.1% required incisional glaucoma surgery.

SECTION 6: RETINAL VEIN OCCLUSIONS
1 CVOS: Central Retinal Vein Occlusion Study (1995)
Aim: to determine whether macular grid laser improves visual outcomes in central retinal vein occlusion (CRVO) and if PRP can prevent neovascularisation if there is greater than 10 DD of retinal ischaemia.
Details: 3-year follow-up, 155 participants. Two arms: macular grid laser section – macular grid laser versus no treatment; PRP section – scatter PRP versus no treatment.
Outcome: there was *no observed difference between final VA in either group*, and preemptive PRP did not prevent neovascularisation.

2 BVOS: Branch retinal Vein Occlusion Study (1984)
Aim: to ascertain if macular grid laser improves visual outcomes in branch retinal vein occlusion (BRVO) with macular oedema and whether PRP can prevent neovascularisation.
Details: 3-year follow-up, 139 participants. Two arms: macular grid laser section – macular grid laser versus no treatment; PRP section – sectoral scatter PRP versus no treatment. Patients had 6/12 vision or worse before macular laser treatment was initiated.
Outcome: macular oedema patients treated with *grid laser were more likely to gain at least two lines of Snellen acuity*, and PRP should be performed only when neovascularisation is detected.

3 CRUISE: Ranibizumab for macular edema following branch retinal vein occlusion (2010)
Aim: to determine the safety and efficacy of intravitreal ranibizumab for macular oedema in patients with CRVO.
Details: 6-month follow-up, 392 participants. Three arms: monthly (1) sham injections, (2) 0.3 mg ranibizumab injections and (3) 0.5 mg ranibizumab injections.
Outcome: *patients receiving ranibizumab did better*, as the 0.3 mg and 0.5 mg doses resulted in an acuity gain of 12.7 and 14.9 letters, respectively, while those receiving sham injections experienced a 0.8 letter gain.

4 BRAVO: Ranibizumab for macular edema following branch retinal vein occlusion (2010)
Aim: to determine the safety and efficacy of intravitreal ranibizumab for macular oedema in patients with BRVO.
Details: 6-month follow-up, 397 participants. Three arms: monthly (1) sham injections, (2) 0.3 mg ranibizumab injections and (3) 0.5 mg ranibizumab injections.
Outcome: *patients receiving ranibizumab did better*, as the 0.3 mg and 0.5 mg doses resulted in an acuity gain of 16.6 and 18.3 letters respectively, while those receiving sham injections experienced a 7.3 letter gain.

5 GENEVA: Randomized, sham-controlled trial of dexamethasone intravitreal implant in patients with macular edema due to retinal vein occlusion (2010)
Aim: to determine the safety and efficacy of a single intravitreal dexamethasone implant in the treatment of BRVO and CRVO.
Details: 6-month follow-up, 1267 participants. Three arms: (1) 0.35 mg dexamethasone implant, (2) 0.7 mg dexamethasone implant and (3) sham implant.
Outcome: both the 0.35 mg and the 0.7 mg *dexamethasone implants were associated with*

greater visual gains than the sham implant, with an IOP of greater than 25 mmHg occurring in 16% of those participants receiving dexamethasone implants.

6 COPERNICUS: Intravitreal Aflibercept Injection for Macular Edema Due to Central Retinal Vein Occlusion (2013)

Aim: this was designed to evaluate the efficacy of intravitreal aflibercept in patients with macular oedema secondary to CRVO.

Details: 1-year follow-up, 189 participants. Two groups: monthly aflibercept for 6 months followed by PRN aflibercept and sham injection followed by PRN aflibercept.

Outcome: those in the *aflibercept group fared better*, with 56.1% experiencing a gain of 15 letters at 6 months, versus 12.3% of those in the sham group, which was maintained at 1 year.

SECTION 7: OTHER EYE STUDIES

1 HEDS I: Herpetic Eye Disease Study I (1996)

Aim: to determine (1) the efficacy of topical corticosteroids with topical trifluridine in treating stromal simplex, these plus oral acyclovir (2) in treating stromal simplex and (3) in treating simplex iridocyclitis.

Details: there were various numbers of participants in the three study groups. In the first, topical steroids versus sham drops (both with trifluridine); the second and third study oral acyclovir versus sham tablets, with all groups receiving topical steroids and trifluridine.

Outcome: topical *steroids hastened the resolution of stromal keratitis* but did not affect the end VA, while the addition of oral acyclovir was of no benefit in stromal simplex but did trend towards significance in treating simplex iridocyclitis.

2 HEDS II: Herpetic Eye Disease Study II (1998)

Aim: to determine (1) the efficacy of oral acyclovir in addition to topical acyclovir in treating epithelial simplex and (2) the preventative effect of oral acyclovir in reducing recurrence rates.

Details: there were different numbers of participants in the two study groups. In the first, oral acyclovir versus sham tablet, both with topical antivirals; in the second, oral acyclovir 400 mg twice daily or placebo for a year.

Outcome: there was no benefit in adding oral acyclovir in epithelial disease, but, in the preventative arm, *oral acyclovir reduced the recurrence rate* of any herpetic disease in the eye by 41% and of stromal disease by 50%.

3 EVS: Endophthalmitis Vitrectomy Study (1995)

Aim: to determine the usefulness of pars plana vitrectomy and systemic steroids in the treatment of endophthalmitis occurring less than 6 weeks following cataract surgery.

Details: 9-month follow-up, 420 eyes. Four arms: (1) vitrectomy or (2) vitreous tap and antibiotics (vancomycin and amikacin), plus either treatment with (3) or without (4) IV antibiotics (amikacin and ceftazidime).

Outcome: systemic antibiotics had no effect on disease progress, while *vitrectomy resulted in a 50% decrease in severe visual loss* and a threefold increase in those achieving 6/12 or better – but only in those with light perception vision at presentation.

4 COMS: Collaborative Ocular Melanoma Study (2001)

Aim: to study the mortality rates in untreated small (1–3 mm thickness, greater than 5 mm diameter) choroidal melanomas, compare survival rates between patients with medium-size tumours (less than 10 mm thickness, less than 16 mm diameter) treated with I-125 brachytherapy and enucleation, and compare survival rates between patients with large-size tumours pretreated with radiotherapy prior to enucleation and those not pretreated.

Details: 5-year follow-up, various numbers of participants in the study groups. Small tumours were simply observed, medium tumours were randomised to brachytherapy or enucleation and large tumours were randomised to pre-enucleation radiotherapy or not. **Outcome:** at 5 years, *small tumours had a mortality of 6% and could be observed,* medium tumours had similar survival rates (82% in the I-125 group vs 81% in the enucleation group) and pre-treating large tumours with radiation did not improve survival (57% for untreated vs 62% for treated).

5 MIVI-TRUST: Trial of Microplasmin IntraVitreal Injection for non-surgical treatment of focal vitreomacular adhesion (2012)

Aim: to assess whether intravitreal ocriplasmin can resolve vitreomacular adhesion in patients with symptomatic macular holes.

Details: 28-day follow-up, 652 participants. Two arms: intravitreal ocriplasmin and sham injection.

Outcome: *vitreomacular adhesion resolved in a slightly higher proportion of ocriplasmin-treated eyes,* at 26.5% versus 10.1% for placebo treated eyes.

Summary of The Royal College of Ophthalmologists, National Institute for Health and Care Excellence, and Driver and Vehicle Licensing Agency guidance

Summary of major Royal College of Ophthalmologists and National Institute for Health and Care Excellence guidelines in Ophthalmology

Authority	Subject area	Guidance

RCOphth	**Diabetic retinopathy: follow-up**	• BDR: annual digital photograph (two field is standard)
		• PPDR: 4–6/12; first-year conversion to PDR = 3.2%
		• High-risk PPDR: first-year conversion to PDR = 48.5%
		• Consider prophylactic PRP in:
		  » older patients with T2DM
		  » prior to phacoemulsification
		  » in the second eye when the first has been lost to PDR
		  » when clinic attendance is likely to be poor

RCOphth	**Diabetic retinopathy laser**	PDR: same day (within 2/52) – full PRP: • 'full' = 4/4 quadrants, pre- and post-equatorial retina to arcades • 0.1–0.5 s × 300–400 µm × 1.5 burn-width spacing. ETDRS-suggested minimum of 236 mm^2 = 1600 burns. Visible as immediate grey/white mark Diabetic vitreous haemorrhage or PDR: consider early vitrectomy

RCOphth	**Diabetic maculopathy**
	Treatment:
	• non-centre-involving CSMO: grid laser
	• centre-involving CSMO and CRT >250:
	  » VA unaffected: laser or observe
	  » VA 78–24 letters, pseudophake: Lucentis® or IVTA ± laser
	  » VA 78–24 letters, phakic: Lucentis
	  » VA <24 letters: observe; can consider Lucentis/IVTA
	  » VMT: vitrectomy ± Lucentis/IVTA
	• non-central or <400: physician's discretion
		CSMO definition (according to the ETDRS):
		• thickening within 500 µm of fovea
		• Hard exudates within 500 µm if associated with adjacent retinal thickening
		• retinal thickening of 1 DD within 1 DD of fovea

RCOphth	**Ocular tumour referral to tertiary centres (Liverpool, Sheffield, London and Glasgow)**	• Refer all intraocular tumours • Refer all conjunctival and epibulbar tumours • Refer conjunctival melanocytic tumours where there are/is:

(Continued)

Authority	Subject area	Guidance

	Ocular tumour referral to tertiary centres (*cont.*)	» involvement of cornea, caruncle or palpebral conjunctiva
		» feeder vessels
		» diffuse pigmentation
		» diameter exceeds 3 mm
		● Refer iris nodules with any of:
		  » >3 mm diameter
		  » elevated tumour
		  » secondary glaucoma or cataract
		  » involving angle

RCOphth	**Retinal vein occlusion**
	
	All patients with retinal vein occlusion should have:
	● a clinical exam:
	  » BCVA
	  » pupils
	  » IOP
	  » gonioscopy
	  » slit lamp
	● retinal imaging:
	  » colour fundus
	  » OCT with Zeiss Stratus or similar
	  » FFA when no significant vitreous haemorrhage
	● systemic investigations:
	  » full blood count and erythrocyte sedimentation rate/plasma viscosity
	  » Us and Es
	  » BM
	  » cholesterol and high-density lipoprotein
	  » plasma protein electrophoresis
	  » electrocardiogram
	  » TFTs
	● also consider testing for:
	  » thrombophilia
	  » anti-cardiolipin/lupus
	  » C-reactive protein
	  » s-ACE
	  » ANA/Rh/ANCA
	  » chest X-ray
	  » homocysteine
	Target levels:
	● BP <140/85
	● cholesterol <4.8
	● HbA1c <7%
	● random glucose >7.0 mmol
		NI-CRVO:
		● VA 6/12 or worse and CRT >250
		  » Ozurdex® (licensed) or PRN ranibizumab (CRUISE study) (unlicensed)
		● brisk RAPD/VA 6/96 or worse
		  » likely ischaemic, no prescription (Rx), await NV
		● retreat unless/until VA better than 6/7.5, CRT <250, or clinician decides to stop
		
		I-CRVO:
		● NVI/NVA with open angle
		  » PRP ± bevacizumab (unlicensed), 6-weekly follow-up with redo if persistent NV
		  » 3-monthly follow-up to 1 year
		● NVI/NVA with closed angle
		  » PRP ± bevacizumab (unlicensed) and referral to glaucoma team for consideration of diode/GDD
		● no anterior-segment NV and regular follow-up impractical: PRP
		
		NI-BRVO:
		● macular oedema:
		  » Ozurdex (licensed) or ranibizumab (unlicensed) if seen within 3 months
		  » if seen after 3/12, Ozurdex (licensed), ranibizumab (unlicensed) or laser
		● retreatment:
		  » retreat unless/until:
		    — VA 6.0/7.5 or better or
		    — CRT <250
		    — clinical decision to stop
		● Ozurdex every 4–6 months
		● ranibizumab monthly for first 6 months then PRN (BRAVO)
		  » grid laser retreatment every 4 months
		
		Hemivein occlusion:
		● risk of macular oedema similar to that with BRVO
		● risk of NV less than that with CRVO and more than that with BRVO

Authority	Subject area	Guidance

NICE	**OHT/(COAG) treatment**
	*Monitor IOP, VF, optic nerve head
	Low-risk: follow-up every 1–2 years
	High-risk: follow-up every 6–12 months
		Suspected COAG:
		• presenting IOP >32, any age, any CCT
		• treat with a prostaglandin analogue
		• presenting IOP 25–32:
		  » CCT 555–590
		    – treat with beta blockers until 60 years old
		    – CCT <555
		  » treat with *PGA* until 80 presenting IOP 21–25:
		  » CCT <555
		  » treat with *PGA* until 60
		  » CCT 555–590
		  » monitor*
		• presenting IOP 21–32:
		  » CCT >590
		  » monitor*
		
		Established COAG: monitor every 2–6 months:
		• advanced disease
		• *augmented surgery*
		• early or moderate disease
		  » Prostaglandin analogue

RCOphth	**ROP**
	Definitions:
	• stage 1: demarcation line
	• stage 2: ridge
	• stage 3: extraretinal fibrovascular proliferation
	• stage 4: subtotal retinal detachment
	  » 4A extrafoveal
	  » 4B foveal
	• stage 5: total RD
	• plus disease: venous dilation and arterial insufficiency compared with a standard photo
	(*See* Figure A.1 ROP zones, p. 129)
		Monitoring intervals:
		• every 2 weeks:
		  » stage 0 in zone II
		  » stage 1 or 2 in zone II or III with no plus
		• weekly:
		  » Stage 0 Vessels in zone I
		  » stage 1 or 2 in zones II or III with pre-plus
		  » stage 1 or 2 in zone I
		  » stage 1 in zone II with plus
		  » stage 3 in zone II or III
		  » any stage in zone III with plus
		• at least weekly:
		  » stage 2 in zone II with plus
		Treatment:
		• consider Rx:
		  » stage 2 in zone II with plus
		• urgent Rx:
		  » any stage in zone I with plus
		  » stage 3 in zone I without plus
		  » stage 3 in zone II with plus

RCOphth	**Device decontamination**	Sterilisation of tonometer heads: 1 keep device moist until decontaminated 2 wash with clean running water and soap 3 soak for 10 minutes in sodium hypochlorite solution (10 000 ppm chlorine) i.e. Milton solution 4 rinse thoroughly with sterile water 5 dry with paper towels and store dry

(Continued)

Authority	Subject area	Guidance
RCOphth	**Device contamination** (*cont.*)	Alcohol wipes fix prion particles and are not recommended for cleaning tonometer heads. Further, 70% alcohol will not clear all virus particles
		College guidance states that disposable heads *may* be used for patients at high risk of Creutzfeldt–Jakob disease (CJD); the use of these is not mandatory in any circumstance
RCOphth/ Department of Health	**CJD risk stratification** **Blood transfusions are only considered high risk if the patient has received more than 80 donors (total of more than 50 units, or transfusions on more than 20 occasions)	Ask the patient: • 'Have you ever been notified that you are at increased risk of CJD or variant CJD?' • 'Have you ever received growth hormone or gonadotrophin treatment?'
	High-risk surgery: • posterior segment/retina Special measures: • instrument quarantine • use disposables • incinerate after use/send to Health Protection Agency storage • GP referral • involve Infectious diseases and Microbiology	• 'Have you ever had surgery on your brain or spinal cord?' • 'Since 1980, have you had any blood products?'** If the patient responds: • no to all: proceed to surgery with standard precautions • yes to any:** increased risk, consider special measures
RCOphth	**Vigabatrin-associated field loss** Vigabatrin is an anti-epileptic used in partial epilepsy, with and without secondary generalisation. It is used as first-line/monotherapy in West's syndrome (infantile spasms). There is less than 1:1000 symptomatic peripheral-field loss and no evidence of continuing visual-field loss after cessation. Risk of vigabatrin-attributed visual-field constriction (VAVFC) is very low when the treatment duration is >5 years or the cumulative dose is >5 kg	Patients able to undertake perimetry: • test before Rx and then at 6 monthly intervals for 5 years then annually if no VAVFC detected: » static suprathreshold to at least 45 degrees of eccentricity (FF120) or kinetic (III-4e/I-4e/I-2e) » when VAVFC detected, repeat to confirm before cessation of drug Patients unable to undertake perimetry (<9 years): • field-specific VEP only alternative • when findings suggest peripheral loss, discuss cessation with patient/parents/carers

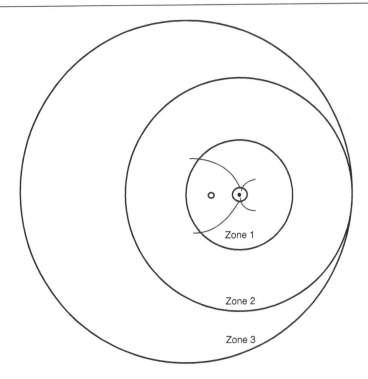

Zone 1 is a circle centred on the disc whose radius is twice the distance from the disc to the fovea
Zone 2 is a circle based on the disc whose radius extends to the nasal ora serrata
Zone 3 is the remaining crescent of temporal retina

FIGURE A.1 ROP zones

Summary of Driver and Vehicle Licensing Agency driving standards (2013): Class 1 licence holders

- VA: in good daylight, with appropriate refractive correction, the patient must be able to read (post 1 September 2001) a number plate from 20 m.
- Visual field: the minimum visual field is at least 120 degrees on the horizontal, measured using a target equivalent to Goldmann III4e; extension should be at least 50 degrees left and right. In addition, there should be no significant defect in the binocular field that encroaches within 20 degrees of fixation above or below the horizontal meridian.
    - ➤ A 'significant central defect' is:
        - — a cluster of four or more adjoining points that is wholly or partly within the central 20 degrees
        - — loss consisting of both a single cluster of three adjoining missed points up to and including the central 20 degrees from fixation and any additional separate missed point(s) within the central 20 degrees
        - — any central loss that is an extension of a hemianopia or quadrantanopia of size greater than three missed points.
- Diplopia: driving must cease on diagnosis. Driving may resume after confirmation from the Driver and Vehicle Licensing Agency that the diplopia is controlled by glasses or by a patch that the licence holder undertakes to wear while driving. A stable, uncorrected diplopia of 6 months' duration or more may be compatible with driving if there is consultant support indicating satisfactory functional adaptation.
- Specific considerations and guidance are issued concerning particular eye diseases – these should be referred to when there is a question of fitness to drive.

Index

Entries in **bold** denote figures.

sub-threshold testing 51
suprachoroidal effusion 74
supra-duction 12
suprathreshold testing 51
suture-tying forceps 75, 79

tarsorrhaphy **95–6**
  permanent 96–7
  temporary 83, 94–6
TBUT (tear-film break-up time) 70–1
Teller Acuity Cards 5, **6**
temporal artery biopsy 41, 102–3, **103**
temporal retina 51, **129**
Tenon's capsule 64
thyroid eye disease 94
tissue perfusion, reduced 40
tonometer heads, sterilisation of 127–8
Tono-Pen **24**
toothed forceps 98
topical anaesthesia
  in applanation tonometry 22
  in fundus examination 30
  in intravitreal injections **58**
  for laser therapy 104–6, 110–12
  in local anaesthesia 60–2, 64
  procedures using 74–6, 78–80, 87–9
  in surgery 61
torsional movements 12–13
total deviation 52
trabeculectomy, studies on 115–16
transillumination defect 76
triamcinolone 121
trifluridine 123
tropias (manifest deviations) 19–20
tropicamide 76
Tube Versus Trabeculectomy Study 116

UBM (ultrasound biomicroscopy) 36, 41
ultrasound
  biometry 46
  biomicroscopy 36
  pachymetry **38**
  techniques of 41–3
United Kingdom Prospective Diabetes Study 120
uveitis 87, 108

Vannas scissors 79
vascular abnormality 39–40
vascular hypoperfusion 40
VAVFC (vigabatrin-attributed visual-field
  constriction) 128
VEGF trap-eye 118
VEP (visual evoked potential) 44–5, 128
vergences, in ocular movement 12
vernier acuity 3
versions, in ocular movement 12, 14
Verteporfin in Photodynamic Therapy
  116
vertical diplopia 16
vertical recti 13, 15–16
Vicryl sutures 93
videokeratoscopy 35
vigabatrin 128
vision, hill of 51
vision charts 3
visual acuity (VA)
  assessment of 3
  notation of 4
visual field
  for driving 129
  testing 51–3
visual loss
  and intravitreal injection 57
  and laser therapy 112
vitamins C and E 118
vitrectomy 120, 123, 125
vitreomacular adhesion 124
vitreous detachments 42–3
vitreous haemorrhage 76, 120, 126
vitreous tap 123
Vogt's striae 35

Westcott scissors 64, **65**, 96
West's syndrome 128
window defects 39–40
WTW (white-to-white) 50

YAG (yttrium aluminium garnet) laser 16,
  104–6, 109–12

zinc 118

CPD with Radcliffe

You can now use a selection of our books to achieve CPD (Continuing Professional Development) points through directed reading.

We provide a free online form and downloadable certificate for your appraisal portfolio. Look for the CPD logo and register with us at: www.radcliffehealth.com/cpd

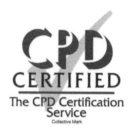